Synthesis Lectures on Human-Centered Informatics

Series Editor

John M. Carroll, College of Information Sciences and Technology, Penn State University, University Park, USA

This series publishes short books on Human-Centered Informatics (HCI), at the intersection of the cultural, the social, the cognitive, and the aesthetic with computing and information technology. Lectures encompass a huge range of issues, theories, technologies, designs, tools, environments, and human experiences in knowledge, work, recreation, and leisure activity, teaching and learning, etc. The series publishes state-of-the-art syntheses, case studies, and tutorials in key areas. It shares the focus of leading international conferences in HCI.

John M. Carroll · Jeongwon Jo · Srishti Gupta ·
Fanlu Gui · Jomara Sandbulte · Ya-Fang Lin ·
Sooyeon Lee · Tiffany Knearem ·
Chun-Hua Tsai

Coproducing Care
Synergies of Recognition

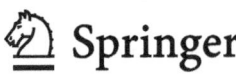

John M. Carroll
College of Information Sciences
and Technology
Pennsylvania State University
University Park, PA, USA

Srishti Gupta
Massry School of Business
State University of New York at Albany
New York, NY, USA

Jomara Sandbulte
Department of Computer Science
University of Minnesota at Duluth
Duluth, MN, USA

Sooyeon Lee
Department of Informatics
New Jersey Institute of Technology
Newark, NJ, USA

Chun-Hua Tsai
Department of Information Systems
and Quantitative Analysis
University of Nebraska at Omaha
Omaha, NE, USA

Jeongwon Jo
Department of Computer Science
and Engineering
University of Notre Dame
Notre Dame, IN, USA

Fanlu Gui
College of Information Sciences
and Technology
Pennsylvania State University
University Park, PA, USA

Ya-Fang Lin
College of Information Sciences
and Technology
Pennsylvania State University
University Park, PA, USA

Tiffany Knearem
College of Information Sciences
and Technology
Pennsylvania State University
University Park, PA, USA

ISSN 1946-7680   ISSN 1946-7699 (electronic)
Synthesis Lectures on Human-Centered Informatics
ISBN 978-3-032-04303-0   ISBN 978-3-032-04304-7 (eBook)
https://doi.org/10.1007/978-3-032-04304-7

© The Editor(s) (if applicable) and The Author(s), under exclusive license to Springer Nature Switzerland AG 2026

This work is subject to copyright. All rights are solely and exclusively licensed by the Publisher, whether the whole or part of the material is concerned, specifically the rights of translation, reprinting, reuse of illustrations, recitation, broadcasting, reproduction on microfilms or in any other physical way, and transmission or information storage and retrieval, electronic adaptation, computer software, or by similar or dissimilar methodology now known or hereafter developed.
The use of general descriptive names, registered names, trademarks, service marks, etc. in this publication does not imply, even in the absence of a specific statement, that such names are exempt from the relevant protective laws and regulations and therefore free for general use.
The publisher, the authors and the editors are safe to assume that the advice and information in this book are believed to be true and accurate at the date of publication. Neither the publisher nor the authors or the editors give a warranty, expressed or implied, with respect to the material contained herein or for any errors or omissions that may have been made. The publisher remains neutral with regard to jurisdictional claims in published maps and institutional affiliations.

This Springer imprint is published by the registered company Springer Nature Switzerland AG
The registered company address is: Gewerbestrasse 11, 6330 Cham, Switzerland

If disposing of this product, please recycle the paper.

Foreword

The closest thing to being cared for is to care for someone else
(McCullers, 1958)

Caring for other people is fundamental to humanity. We care for family members, such as children and parents, creating and strengthening the bonds of family. We care for neighbors and fellow citizens, building solidarity and community. We encourage others, and we convey appreciation for what they do. We comfort others; we actively listen, and we hold hands. We engage with others in personal activities like cooking, cleaning, and shopping, and in community activities such as food sharing and neighborhood safety.

Society facilitates and regulates a wide range of more formal caring interactions, including personal services like hair styling and manicure, educational services like schools and apprenticeships, health services like massage and nutrition guidance, medical services like nursing and hospitals, and so forth.

All this caring does not mean that we fully understand how care works, or that we currently deploy and benefit from care in all the right ways. As an example of the contrary, in the United States some analysts complain that medical institutions achieve poor care outcomes and cost too much (Crowley et al., 2020). Others complain that unpaid care work can be a burden, valued in billions of dollars annually, that falls disproportionately on mothers and daughters in traditional families (Jacoby et al., 2024). Significant research on caregiving also sadly shows that it can be a stressful activity, and that many caregivers, paid and unpaid, eventually suffer burnout (Lynch & Lobo, 2012).

Here my co-authors and I attempt to move beyond the economic paradigm of receiving or delivering care to the joint activity of creating and sharing care. Although care often is succinctly received or delivered and formally compensated, in other cases it is volunteered and coproduced. Coproduced care is reciprocally exchanged and acknowledged; everyone involved participates and experiences social and emotional benefits. Participants feel cared for, supported, and safe, but also competent, efficacious, and powerful. Moreover, each participant feels and can appreciate that the others are directly contributing to these beneficial experiences.

A minimal example is the contrast between a woman receiving a manicure from another woman, and two teenage girls giving manicures to one another. The first case is one of delivery and receipt; the participants play distinct roles; indeed, one pays the other to receive a service. The second case is one of creating and sharing reciprocal care and acknowledgment. Both girls learn about and experience manicure, as well as about caring for others.

More complex scenarios involve people creating everyday care synergies through reciprocal coproduction, for example, a younger depressed person accompanies an older person who lives alone on a shopping trip. The depressed person contributes to the project, experiencing concrete self-efficacy and self-worth. The older person receives concrete shopping assistance and social support.

Such an interaction challenges conventional economic views of care: Both participants might come away feeling that they received and experienced care, but neither might feel that they provided care per se. Yet, from a societal standpoint, one participant received clinical care for depression and the other received elder care for independent living; in many countries, both kinds are provided by government-financed programs (Glynos & Speed, 2012).

In this book, we explore and discuss the coproduction of care as an obvious everyday paradigm for caring that is, at the same time, often invisible.

We are very grateful to Prof. Airi Lampinen for comments on an earlier draft.

State College, PA, USA
June 2025

Jack Carroll

References

Crowley, R., Daniel, H., Cooney, T. G., Engel, L. S., Health and Public Policy Committee of the American College of Physicians* (2020). Envisioning a better US health care system for all: Coverage and cost of care. *Annals of Internal Medicine, 172*(2_Supplement), S7–S32.

Glynos, J., & Speed, E. (2012). Varieties of co-production in public services: Time banks in a UK health policy context. *Critical Policy Studies, 6*(4), 402–433.

Jacoby, A., Sen, A., Kelley, G., & Montoya-Boyer, A. (2024). *Unseen work, unmet needs: Exploring the intersections of gender, race and ethnicity in unpaid care labor and paid labor in the US* (tech. rep.). Oxfam America.

Lynch, S. H., & Lobo, M. L. (2012). Compassion fatigue in family caregivers: A wilsonian concept analysis. *Journal of Advanced Nursing, 68*(9), 2125–2134.

McCullers, C. (1958). *The square root of wonderful*. Houghton: Mifflin.

Contents

1 **Introduction** 1
   1.1 Care 1
   1.2 Coproduction 3
   1.3 Additive and Transformative Coproduction 6
   1.4 Salutogenic Care 9
   References 11

2 **Coproducing Care in Everyday Life** 13
   2.1 Coproducing Care Within Families 15
       2.1.1 Demands for Independence in Traditional Family Care
             Dynamics 15
       2.1.2 Conflicts in Health Beliefs Within Traditional Family Care 17
   2.2 Coproducing Care Between New Parents 18
       2.2.1 Challenges in Task Distribution and Values in Recognizing
             Efforts 18
       2.2.2 Navigating Disagreements and Finding Common Goals 19
   2.3 People with Different Abilities Coproducing Care Through
       Collaborative Shopping 20
       2.3.1 Recognizing Capabilities for Transformative Coproduction 20
   2.4 Coproducing Care and Environmental Health Through
       Community-Based Monitoring 22
       2.4.1 Additive and Transformative Citizen Science 22
       2.4.2 Hackathon to Share Stakes and Transform Roles
             of Stakeholders 23
       2.4.3 Citizen-Based Water Monitoring Increasing Synergies in Local
             Communities 24

	2.5	Coproducing Care Through Community Appreciation	25
		2.5.1 Lack of Visibility to Local Non-profit Groups	25
		2.5.2 Thank-You Station for Coproducing Care Between Volunteers and Local Members	25
	2.6	Coproducing Community Care and Resilience Towards Prolonging Crises	27
		2.6.1 Additive Coproduction of Disaster Relief: Filling in the Gaps in Formal Disaster Response	28
		2.6.2 Transformative Coproduction of Disaster Relief: Citizens and Marginalized Populations as Support Providers	29
		2.6.3 Care Cannot be Automatically Delivered	30
		2.6.4 Benefits of Coproducing Disaster Relief: Increased Collective Resilience and the Role of Visibility	30
		2.6.5 Benefits of Transformative Disaster Relief: Collective Actualization	32
	2.7	Sharing Knowledge as a Form of Care in a Hobbyist Community	32
		2.7.1 Initiating and Joining Beer Brewing Activities	33
	References	35
3	**Discussion**		39
	3.1	Coproducing Care is a Good Way to Work	39
	3.2	The Spectrum of Coproduction	41
	3.3	Synergy as a Defining Characteristic of Coproduction	44
	3.4	Future Implications	45
		3.4.1 Making Different Stakes Salient	46
		3.4.2 Making Contributions Visible	47
		3.4.3 Making Better Use of Resources	49
	3.5	Limitations and Future Work	50
	3.6	Conclusion	52
	References	52

Introduction

A traditional way of thinking about care is as a nuanced variety of service provision. In this view, a person cares for another person through comforting and protecting, through nurturing and sustaining. Friends and family provide care in this sense; health and medical professionals provide care. More broadly, neighbors, co-workers, and fellow citizens provide care; public institutions like schools and social service agencies also provide care.

The spectrum of caring is vast, ranging from informal acts of compassion and acknowledgement throughout daily life, to more focused caring about the welfare of others through teaching and learning, and management of infrastructure, to intimate and lifelong parental and spousal relationships, to the intensive interactions of medical therapies and palliative care.

1.1 Care

Contemporary philosophical consideration of care has emphasized broad ethical and political perspectives, developing out of Mayeroff's (1971) care ethics. Tronto (1993) considered care a central activity of human life that focuses on ethical responsibilities of remaining in, continuing, and repairing the world. She argued that society has undervalued care provision to preserve the status quo of power and privilege, and that lower-status people have often been oppressed with burdens of care provision. She analyzed care provision into four types or stages: recognizing that care is needed, taking responsibility for the need, care provision, the response to receiving care. de La Bellacasa (2017) expanded consideration to include human care for all the life and all the material of planet Earth. This led her to transform Tronto's notion of ethical burden in care provision into the political notion that the recipient (organic or inorganic) should be afforded "a careful reciprocity" to "question when and how" care is accepted (de La Bellacas, 2017, p. 120).

Both of these discussions are usefully provocative, but both are quite normative. Tronto suggests that care provision should be more broadly and openly valued and exercised by humans. Yet her view of care is naively unbalanced: almost all agency resides with the caregiver, even though care interactions often fail when care recipients decline care (Cahn, 2000). Puig de la Bellacasa suggests that care is entangled with human interactions in the material world and that humans must be attentive as to whether and how they impose care. This is an insight, but does not go far enough in imagining possible contributions from care recipients in enabling and shaping care interactions. In trying to be fundamental and general about human morality, these positions regard people as generic actors in generic circumstances.

Care ethics conceives of care as a one-directional service provision. It does not imagine possibilities of nuance or synergy in moral conduct, yet recent decades have been morally turbulent. The iconic caring profession of nursing, for example, has transformed itself, professionalizing its role in medical services, embracing the emerging concept of patient-centered care (the expectation that patients can be active participants in their own care) and confronting the relentless challenges of long-term stress for caregivers (Ernst & Tatli, 2022; Shohani & Zamanzadeh, 2017).

Our home "inter-discipline", Human-Computer Interaction (HCI), provides many examples of how care and caring are matters for rethinking and innovation. Our research community of computer scientists, designers, social scientists, and others produces a couple thousand research papers on care per year (an increase of about 7x through the past decade). We identified and examined a sample of 45 so-called full papers (meaning they ranged from 7000–9000 words with about 70–90 citations to scientific literature) published 2022–2024 in the proceedings of premier ACM (Association for Computing Machinery) venues, CHI (the Conference on Computer Human Interaction, 18 papers) and CSCW (the Conference on Computer Supported Cooperative Work, 27 papers). The papers examine the role of innovation and technology in care provision; and present new approaches, studies of people engaging new approaches, or both.

About half of the papers (n = 24) reported on the appropriation and effectiveness of new technological tools and approaches, including interactive 3-D simulations, real time surveillance, computer mediated care interactions between humans, collaborative augmented reality activities, conversational agents, social robots, generative deep learning, machine learning models, human-AI interactions, data-driven care management, customizable clinical dashboards, and self-care technologies. The balance of the papers (21) examined human issues arising in care contexts, such as family coordination and resilience, boundary negotiation, specific care needs, gaps in chronic care management, conflicts and resolution in differing care values and practices, and the use of laboratory test results throughout care trajectories, often through interviews and co-design with care recipients and caregivers.

The papers addressed a diverse range of challenging care contexts and concerns, including food assistance programs managed by municipal government, home health monitoring for older adults, use of breast pumps in the workplace, construction of mental illness narratives online, pediatric and adult cancer, asthma, intimate partner violence, perioperative hypotension, pregnancy, diabetes, epilepsy, dementia, bipolar disorder, autism, severe spinal injury, polycystic ovary syndrome (PCOS), chronic obstructive pulmonary disease (COPD), attention deficit/hyperactivity disorder (ADHD), palliative care, and complications of accessibility, patient legal status and patient compliance/noncompliance with care.

These 45 papers comprise an impressive contribution to understanding and advancing the provision of care. They emphasize concretely how central care is to human life, how technology and social context can differentiate and materialize care provision, and how society can marshal diverse resources, skills and perspectives to rethink and innovate how people receive care. However, it is noteworthy that these articles investigated the care provision that occurs in organizational contexts, mostly within or supervised by medical institutions. Three of the 45 papers were non-medical, examining care in school settings (social robots used by special educators caring for children with autism), care administration in a municipal government office, and the use of breast pumps in workplace contexts, respectively. Care in medical institutions is an important category of care, but caring interactions also play important roles in other formal contexts, as well as in less formal contexts such as family and civic life.

1.2 Coproduction

In some caring interactions, there is a clear distinction between caregivers and care recipients. For example, a person might be institutionalized to receive comprehensive medical care that could include assistance with basic functions like feeding and breathing. Such *custodial care* can be a straightforward service provision; the caregiver is a medical professional, and the person being cared for, who may have severe incapacities, receives care from the professional (Rockwell, 2012; Smith, 1965).

In other cases, care interactions are more subtle and complex in that people receiving care play an active and often essential role in the production of care. For example, teachers provide care to students, but they can only succeed if their students reciprocate by playing an active role by trying to learn. Characterizing teaching as a service that teachers provide and for which students are recipients discounts the essential active reciprocity involved in teaching and learning. Thus, teachers can initiate a kind of care, but it only works when students join the effort. Most family and community care also works like this.

This paradigm of care is quite different from how we understand custodial or professional care. Recall Tronto's (1993) analysis in which the person providing care is entirely responsible for recognizing a need, determining what to do about the need, and then for providing care. The person receiving care remains passive throughout, finally responding to care that was provided.

Elinor Ostrom and Edgar Cahn used the concept of *coproduction* to refer to relationships of essential active reciprocity (including generalized reciprocity). Thus, Ostrom (1996) described how government support services can be more effective when citizens actively participate in the production of those services. Ostrom referred to such arrangements as the coproduction of social goods. Cahn (2000) argued that community-level support services can be more effective when communities facilitate the caring contributions of *all* members of the community, in particular those of marginalized members who could otherwise be seen primarily as people in need of care.

Ostrom (1978, 1996) described a surprising example in which the effectiveness of policing and community safety in Chicago during the 1970s was seen to decline when officers switched from walking neighborhood beats to patrolling in cars. Patrol cars were expected to enhance policing by helping police to cover more territory and to be able to respond faster and farther. As Ostrom noted, this efficiency analysis ignores the benefits that derive from police interacting with citizens in the street, incidentally exchanging information and building mutual trust. Sharing these resources helped police and local citizens to better coproduce community safety (Peyton, 2019); patrol cars undermined that crucial relationship.

Cahn (2000) argued that acknowledging and leveraging the capacities of all members of a community is a key to creating effective care throughout a community. One implementation of this idea, developed in the UK National Health System (NHS), is to incorporate service in a community timebank into therapies for mild depression (Glynos & Speed, 2012). Patients who provided care to others, through phone calls and visits, and help with shopping chores, themselves experienced some relief from depression. In these scenarios, reciprocal caregiving provided care to all.

Coproduction of care is a kind of collaboration, but it is more than a matter of effectively allocating and coordinating work among participants. In Ostrom's example, the police and citizens were not explicitly working together on community safety. The police were working on community safety, but the citizens were merely going about their daily business and activity. They incidentally encounter police officers, come to know them better and eventually interact with them. In Cahn's example, none of the participants are directly working on the project of addressing or easing symptoms of depression; Cahn's timebankers were just chatting and carrying small practical favors for and with one another.

One way that coproduction emerges from such incidental collaborations is that the participants have a variety of roles or stakes in the collaboration; they bring diverse goals and resources. Everyone involved has an interest in the interaction, but not the same interest. In addition, the motivations of various participants can evolve over the course of the interaction. Initially, Ostrom's police officers are walking a beat to ensure local safety, and the citizens incidentally see a police uniform in their streets. Cahn's timebankers are earning and spending time credits, and may also see themselves as participating in community through their timebanking interactions. But after relationships are established, the participants can

1.2 Coproduction

be motivated as well by reciprocal caring, empathy and acknowledgment operating at a more personal level. That is to say, the participants come to see one another as particular people they know and with whom they interact.

It is notable and important that coproduction enables synergistic collective outcomes. Something more than the sum of the contributions emerges. In Ostrom's example, the involvement of the citizens in their own policing enhances their engagement and empowerment with respect to community safety. These are separate positive social outcomes, distinct from the objective enhancement of community safety, though it is likely that the social benefits of working together and improved crime statistics mutually reinforce each other. From the perspective of police, their original goal of community safety is enhanced, but they also build social capital with the community to support future cooperation when they need it. Indeed, looking at Ostrom's example counter-factually, the costs of police and citizens *not* building social capital through the course of policing can be quite high for all concerned.

Cahn's example also illustrates striking synergies. The smallish personal services exchanged through timebanks, and officially regulated by time dollars, are a vehicle for building community, one tie at a time. A key synergy in Cahn's timebanking approach is that volunteer time is both free and immeasurably valuable. In the NHS depression scenarios, the participants are chatting and carrying out errands, lightweight interactions that are nevertheless recognized as having value in timebanking. Through this lightweight activity, participants are building interpersonal connections, and also building views of themselves as efficacious and caring people, based on the evidence of their own interactions. One participant gains time dollars and the other spends time dollars, but both see concretely how they can be effective participants in caring interactions.

The care paradigm of coproduction can seem oddly disconnected from recent care ethics scholarship in the humanities, such as Tronto and de la Bellacasa, and from the sociotechnical research in HCI, such as the 45 papers we examined. Indeed, neither Ostrom nor Cahn are cited in these literatures. (Note that Ostrom's work on commoning and the tragedy of the commons, and Cahn's work on timebanks are well recognized in other sociotechnical contexts). The reason for this disconnect appears to be that care ethics has focused on normative care imperatives and not on individual initiative and innovation in interpersonal care; it addresses caring responsibilities, but not actual caring interactions. Sociotechnical care research focuses on care innovation, but often within organizational contexts that strictly distinguish caregivers from care recipients. This implicitly frames interpersonal innovations, especially those of care recipients, as incidental to caring.

When care interactions are constituted by active and reciprocal participation of caregivers and care recipients in innovative and synergistic care exchange, it makes sense to acknowledge this in terminology. Here we use the role terms *initiators* and *joiners* to emphasize the joint activity that constitutes coproduced caring interactions (Carroll et al., 2016), but also to distinguish coproduced care from custodial stereotypes of what care can be.

In this short book, we review studies of informal caring interactions to identify and analyze how care is coproduced in a variety of daily-life contexts. We consider family members discussing healthy behaviors, parents raising their children together, people with different abilities shopping together, an environmental community group that measures water quality, community members acknowledging contributions of fellow community members, and local hobbyists sharing and developing craft knowledge. In reflecting on these cases together we hope to more broadly understand how and with what consequences interpersonal caring interactions are coproduced, and how such coproduction might be more deliberately facilitated through research practices and designs.

We hope our discussion of this work can be of broad use in care discourses and practices. The absence of Ostrom and Cahn from care ethics and sociotechnical research is worrying and limiting, yet across the world, synergies of reciprocity in care are becoming increasingly well-known. For example, the British NHS practice of prescribing service in timebanks for depression (Glynos & Speed, 2012) has expanded greatly in Britain and to several other countries, where it is sometimes now referred to as social prescribing (Moffatt et al., 2023). As we write this in early 2025, the Big Brothers, Big Sisters of America, a large mentoring-oriented nonprofit organization that supports children, emphasized in an interview with US National Public Radio that mentoring relationships typically benefit the person being mentored as well as the mentor.

1.3 Additive and Transformative Coproduction

Coproduction has resonated in many contemporary disciplines and literatures ranging from healthcare to public administration. This breadth of impact itself suggests the broad importance of the concept, and of better understanding and applying it. Not surprisingly, the term is not always used in the same way. Here we focus on Cahn and Ostrom, who helped to initially frame coproduction, but framed it somewhat differently from one another (Glynos & Speed, 2012) and impacted somewhat different disciplines.

In both Cahn's and Ostrom's views of coproduction, human synergies are realized through cooperation. Ostrom's relatively *additive* view of coproduction focuses on synergies of leveraging insights, efforts, and resources of different constituencies, specifically, government workers and the public. In her view, more diverse insight, effort, and resourcing is better. When diverse individuals participate together in a significant human activity, they do not change their social constituencies or community roles. Government workers remain government workers, and citizens are still citizens. But each constituency understands the other better, and they understand how they can serve the needs of communities better together. The public system - for example, the local policing system - is transformed; police and citizens cooperate, negotiate, and exchange insights and perspectives. Through this, they become more knowledgeable and empathetic and more interdependent on one another. Together they coproduce better community policing.

1.3 Additive and Transformative Coproduction

Cahn's more *transformative* view of coproduction focuses on the synergies of recognizing capacity and possibility in others; especially in those who are marginal in various senses. This recognition is a personally and often reciprocally transformative experience. By definition, it is not the way things typically work; if it were, there would be no marginal people. Recognizing capacities and possibilities in others immediately changes the range of roles people can play, what they can mean to us, and the interactions and experiences we can share with them. The NHS example shows how subtle such transformations can be. Two people acknowledging the value of one another can simultaneously enable and evoke care for each of them. When many individuals engage in such coproduction, as in a timebank exchange system, this transformation can be collectivized through institutions, such as the local community.

Ostrom's view of coproduction is an insight into efficiency, effectiveness, and satisfaction with services. Cahn's view is more radical in that social values such as equality, reciprocity, and participation are not only prerequisites for coproduction but animating goals and benefits of coproduction. Recognizing another person's value is not just a step toward caregiving, it is the key step toward being part of the coproduction of care. Importantly, the two streams of research, policy and innovation on coproduction are distinguishable but not contradictory (Glynos & Speed, 2012).

Public administration and health and wellness are two domains that have broadly appropriated coproduction. In public administration, theoretical work has focused on levels of analysis, phases of the service cycle, centrality to institutional mission, and the extent to which coproduction is voluntary (Brandsen & Honingh, 2016; Brudney & England, 1983; Nabatchi et al., 2017). This literature tends to point to Ostrom as a single point of origin. This makes sense in that Ostrom herself focused on dynamics in citizen relationships with government. Ostrom tended to prioritize the voluntarily initiated coordination of embodied practices toward concrete results consistent with extant institutional objectives, as in the example of policing in Chicago.

Subsequent work in public administration articulated a broader space of coproduction relationships. With respect to levels of analysis, this work distinguished among cases in which individual actors coproduce a result (a doctor and patient work together on implementing a program of dietary and exercise interventions), groups coproduce a result (a collection of school officials, teachers, and parents of children with special needs work together to provide in-class and after school educational activities), and institutions participate in coproducing a result (a local parks department works with citizens to construct and manage a network of bicycle routes; examples drawn from Nabatchi et al., 2017).

With respect to phases of the service cycle, this work distinguished among cases of co-commissioning (a doctor and patient work together to identify and prioritize health issues), co-design (a doctor and patient plan to address health issues), co-delivery (a doctor and patient implement a program of dietary and exercise interventions), and co-assessment (a doctor and patient evaluate their interventions; examples drawn from Nabatchi et al., 2017).

Each phase of the service cycle can be crossed with each level of analysis, resulting in $3 \times 4 = 12$ canonical types of service coproduction. Nabatchi et al. (2017) note that this typology affords more precise consideration of how participants are motivated and can be incentivized to engage in various types of coproduction, how management and leadership issues vary across types of coproduction, in what circumstances various types should be engaged and with what expected outcomes, and so forth.

Articulating the space of coproduction relationships and phases of the service cycle shows how both direct and generalized reciprocity constitute coproduction. For example, a doctor and patient, a teacher and a student, and a parks official and a bicycle hobbyist reciprocate directly within a caring coproduction. In a particular interaction, direct reciprocity is critical, and the social service professional might typically be the initiator. However, the patient, the student or the cyclist could also be an initiator, and their social service partner could be the joiner. At higher levels of analysis, reciprocity can be generalized; an episode of citizen engagement enhances the engagement of all citizens in the bicycle route, and changes the broader relationship between the parks department and local citizens.

The taxonomic focus of public administration research on implementations of additive coproduction provides templates for engaging citizens in government and other institutional work. This advances Ostrom's original program, though it can submerge the role of synergy, so vivid in the Chicago policing example, in these coproductions.

A significant impact of coproduction in healthcare is the rationale and adoption of *patient centered* approaches (Palumbo, 2016). Healthcare is a particularly interesting application domain in that both additive and transformative coproduction concepts are engaged, though often not distinguished (Glynos & Speed, 2012). Coproduction in healthcare can emphasize patient choice, such as allowing patients to choose clinicians and hospitals, insurance schemes, etc. Such initiatives are often framed as reformative and/or empowering. But it is also important to note that patient choice is an active contribution that frames a caring interaction, it is not constitutive of the caring interaction. The patient could choose to be treated as an object of care, and play no active role in coproducing care itself.

A stronger paradigm for healthcare coproduction is directly interviewing patients to configure the care interaction, that is, allowing reciprocal initiative from patients within clinical processes, ensuring that patients' felt concerns are discussed, and engaging patients in clinical activities. This is a more engaged role than patient choice, in that patients are allowed and expected to make sustained and active contributions to the planning and execution of their own care.

A third paradigm for coproduction in healthcare requires equitable and reciprocal contributions by patients and clinicians *throughout the caring interaction*. This is transformative coproduction in that it deliberately reconceives the stakeholder roles of patient and clinician. In this paradigm, clinicians and patients make a continuing commitment to share control and responsibility with one another. To fully succeed, both patients and clinicians must experience effective, acknowledged, and trusting collective effort. In Cahn's terms, this involves moving patients from the margins of care interactions to the center through acknowledgment and active utilization by clinicians of the critical capacities and contributions that only patients can provide.

This highest level of patient engagement and agency in healthcare coproductions is obviously more demanding for both clinicians and patients, and even more so because it is a radical departure from institutionalized expectations. In fact, this degree of clinical reciprocity might not be realistic or even permissible in some circumstances of custodial care.

1.4 Salutogenic Care

Ostrom and Cahn emphasized the importance of reciprocal agency in care: the recipient can contribute more and benefit more than just avoid pain and distress, and the provider can do more than just discharge a moral responsibility. Coproducing care makes caring a participatory activity of mutual respect and a context for human development. Thinking about care as a participatory and developmental coproduction raises the question of what kind of need is required to evoke caring.

Tronto's (1993) conception of care hinges on recognition, responsibility-taking, and intervention implementation, all targeted at a need. Many examples of custodial and professional care are evoked in fact by dramatic care needs involving cancer and other major diseases, serious physical injury, behavioral disorders, etc. Obviously, care can be motivated by life-threatening needs. But should this be regarded as a necessary antecedent for care, that is, inherent to all care, or is life-threatening need just one context for care, among others?

Antonovsky (1991) criticized the tendency of clinicians and researchers to regard health as primarily about illness, and to regard good health as essentially the absence of illness. Antonovsky found this to be ironic and inadequate. He conceptualized health as a broad spectrum of states ranging from shimmering vitality to dire suffering, and suggested that research and clinical attention should be distributed across this entire spectrum. It is important to understand disease, disorder, and injury, and to relieve suffering. But it is also important to understand how good health can be strengthened and developed into better health.

Antonovsky proposed a program of salutogenetic research on the nature and achievement of heathiness to complement the established paradigm of pathogenetic health science. For example, he investigated the sense of coherence as a capacity people cultivate to move toward health throughout life, as Antonovsky put it. Sense of coherence incorporates the belief that challenges can be understood, the motivation to deal with challenges, and the summoning and deployment of resources to cope. Sense of coherence and extensions of the concept of coherence to collectives including the family and the community have been researched; for example, sense of coherence appears to strengthen resilience (Lindstrom & Eriksson, 2006).

Antonovsky's (1996) work is part of a broader humanistic movement in social science, and psychology in particular, toward understanding how people can become more healthy, self-aware, empathetic, thoughtful and creative throughout life (Bandura, 1997; Maslow, 1943; Ryan & Deci, 2000).

In this book, we explore the concept of care from the perspective of salutogenesis, in contrast to the traditional view that care is primarily an ameliorative response to deficiencies, such as health issues. Salutogenesis acknowledges the inevitability of stressors and challenges in life, yet emphasizes that all people naturally move towards healthiness, resilience, and autonomy (Antonovsky, 1991). It recognizes individuals' capacity and inclination to care for one another and to continually foster and expand their own well-being as part of everyday life.

We do see care as a moral response to significant human needs, including what Maslow called deficiency needs. But care is much more than this. Like Antonovsky, we feel that focusing exclusively or even primarily on deficiency needs is inadequate. The spectrum of typical care scenarios in human life includes care that helps people thrive, not merely survive; it includes care that legitimizes, acknowledges, and strengthens all human strengths, not merely ameliorating weaknesses and deprivation. Care includes care for everyday mundane problems, such as boredom, overuse of television or social media and for piano arrangements that are too difficult.

Importantly, care includes helping other people enrich their lives, such as achieving and sustaining intimate relationships, and appreciating and participating in artistic and other creative activity. Maslow talked about these as higher needs or growth needs. Such achievements do not arise from a caregiver easing deficiencies so much as from a person recognizing and appropriating opportunities for self-growth. The care role of other people in supporting such achievements is coproduction: Other people can help a person recognize and prioritize self-growth, but they cannot deliver self-growth. The only path to self-growth is self-initiative.

Broadening our conception of care also eases issues in caregiving that depend on accepting a narrower view. For example, seeing care only as a response to deficiency makes accepting care an implicit declaration of incompetence and a social marker of dependence (Lee, 1997, 2002). This can lead people to resist accepting care (Lampinen, 2021). It can undermine the possibility of productive and reciprocal human connections by exaggerating concerns about appearances of power and independence, about imposing burdens on caregivers, and about one's ability to reciprocate care (DePaulo & Fisher, 1980; Lampinen et al. 2013; Lee1997).

Negative self-perceptions of support from others and feelings of burdening and debt should be seen as care pathologies. They are side effects of the simplistic economics of care that does not acknowledge or make use of the synergies of reciprocity evoked in caring interactions. The next chapter presents example cases of coproduced salutogenetic care, illustrating how individuals collectively engaged in mutual care within families for overall well-being and childcare and within neighborhoods to protect local water quality, volunteering, disaster relief, food security, and beer-brewing events. We explore how additive and transformative coproduction dynamics enabled care where custodial care fell short.

References

Antonovsky, A. (1991). The structural sources of salutogenic strengths.

Antonovsky, A. (1996). The salutogenic model as a theory to guide health promotion. *Health Promotion International, 11*(1), 11–18.

Bandura, A. (1997). Self-efficacy: The exercise of control. Macmillan.

Brandsen, T., & Honingh, M. (2016). Distinguishing different types of coproduction: A conceptual analysis based on the classical definitions. *Public Administration Review, 76*(3), 427–435.

Brudney, J. L., & England, R. E. (1983). Toward a definition of the coproduction concept. *Public Administration Review,* 59–65.

Cahn, E. S. (2000). No more throw-away people: The co-production imperative.

Carroll, J. M., Chen, J., Yuan, C. W. T., & Hanrahan, B. V. (2016). In search of coproduction: Smart services as reciprocal activities. *Computer, 49*(7), 26–32.

de La Bellacasa, M. P. (2017). Matters of care: Speculative ethics in more than human worlds (vol. 41). U of Minnesota Press.

DePaulo, B. M., & Fisher, J. D. (1980). The costs of asking for help. *Basic and Applied Social Psychology, 1*(1), 23–35.

Ernst, J., & Tatli, A. (2022). Knowledge legitimacy battles in nursing, quality in care, and nursing professionalization. *Journal of Professions and Organization, 9*(2), 188–201.

Glynos, J., & Speed, E. (2012). Varieties of co-production in public services: Time banks in a uk health policy context. *Critical Policy Studies, 6*(4), 402–433.

Lampinen, A. (2021). The trouble with sharing: Interpersonal challenges in peer- to-peer exchange. Morgan & Claypool Publishers.

Lampinen, A., Lehtinen, V., Cheshire, C., & Suhonen, E. (2013). Indebtedness and reciprocity in local online exchange. In *Proceedings of the 2013 Conference on Computer Supported Cooperative Work* (pp. 661–672).

Lee, F. (1997). When the going gets tough, do the tough ask for help? help seeking and power motivation in organizations. *Organizational Behavior and Human Decision Processes, 72*(3), 336–363.

Lee, F. (2002). The social costs of seeking help. *The Journal of Applied Behavioral Science, 38*(1), 17–35.

Lindström, B., & Eriksson, M. (2006). Contextualizing salutogenesis and antonovsky in public health development. *Health Promotion International, 21*(3), 238–244.

Maslow, A. H. (1943). A theory of human motivation. *Psychological Review, 50*(4), 370.

Mayeroff, M. (1971). *On caring.* Harper & Row.

Moffatt, S., Wildman, J., Pollard, T. M., Gibson, K., Wildman, J. M., O Brien, N., Griffith, B., Morris, S. L., Moloney, E., Jeffries, J., et al. (2023). Impact of a social prescribing intervention in North East England on adults with type 2 diabetes: The spring ne multimethod study. *Public Health Research, 11*(2).

Nabatchi, T., Sancino, A., & Sicilia, M. (2017). Varieties of participation in public services: The who, when, and what of coproduction. *Public Administration Review, 77*(5), 766–776.

Ostrom, E. (1978). Citizen participation and policing: What do we know? *Journal of Voluntary Action Research, 7*(1–2), 102–108.

Ostrom, E. (1996). Crossing the great divide: Coproduction, synergy, and development. *World Development, 24*(6), 1073–1087.

Palumbo, R. (2016). Contextualizing co-production of health care: A systematic literature review. *International Journal of Public Sector Management, 29*(1), 72–90.

Peyton, K., Sierra-Arévalo, M., & Rand, D. G. (2019). A field experiment on community policing and police legitimacy. *Proceedings of the National Academy of Sciences, 116*(40), 19894–19898.

Rockwell, J. (2012). From person-centered to relational care: Expanding the focus in residential care facilities. *Journal of Gerontological Social Work, 55*(3), 233–248.

Ryan, R. M., & Deci, E. L. (2000). Self-determination theory and the facilitation of intrinsic motivation, social development, and well-being. *American Psychologist, 55*(1), 68.

Shohani, M., & Zamanzadeh, V. (2017). Nurses attitude towards professionalization and factors influencing it. *Journal of Caring Sciences, 6*(4), 345.

Smith, D. E. (1965). The logic of custodial organization. *Psychiatry, 28*(4), 311–323.

Tronto, J. (1993). Moral boundaries: A political argument for an ethic of care. Routledge.

Coproducing Care in Everyday Life

In this chapter, we explore seven empirical case studies from different spheres of everyday life that illuminate how care is coproduced through reciprocal interactions. These cases, drawn from our research in the northeastern United States between 2018 and 2024, span family relationships, community initiatives, and hobby groups. While varied in their specific contexts, these cases collectively demonstrate how coproduction can transform traditional care relationships and generate synergistic benefits for all participants. Each one illuminates a dimension of care that goes beyond addressing human deficiency. Together, they help us reconceptualize care as not only a moral response to urgent needs—as Maslow's concept of deficiency needs might suggest—but as a generative force that enables thriving, creativity, and growth.

Each case illustrates distinct aspects of care coproduction while revealing common patterns in how reciprocal caring relationships develop and evolve. Our studies examine: intergenerational family care dynamics; co-parenting relationships; collaborative shopping between people with different abilities; community-based environmental monitoring; mutual aid during crisis; volunteer appreciation; and knowledge sharing in hobby communities. Through these diverse examples, we analyze both additive and transformative forms of coproduction, showing how care relationships can simultaneously strengthen existing social bonds while creating new possibilities for mutual support and growth. Table 2.1 summarizes each case study's context, methodology, manifestations of additive and transformative coproduction, and coproduction outcomes.

The cases were selected to showcase coproduction across different scales of social organization, ranging from intimate family units to broader community networks. Each case employed qualitative research methods including interviews, participant observation, and

Table 2.1 Overview of case studies

Case study	Context	Methodology	Coproduction type	Coproduction outcome
Family Health Care (Sandbulte et al., 2021)	Intergenerational health communication and support between elderly parents and adult children	Focus groups with scenario-based interviews	Additive (health support) and transformative (role redefinition)	Shows challenges in transforming traditional care hierarchies
Co-parenting (Lin et al., 2024)	New parents' collaboration and mutual support strategies	Interview study	Additive (supportive environment) and transformative (relationship evolution)	Demonstrates how reciprocal care strengthens parental bonds and also relationship bonds
Collaborative Shopping (Lee et al., 2020)	Shopping practices between people with visual impairments and sighted companions	Observational case study	Additive (task completion) and transformative (role equality)	Shows how different abilities contribute to shared tasks
Community Water Monitoring	Citizen-based environmental monitoring and stewardship	Hackathon style workshops	Additive (data collection) and transformative (community engagement)	Demonstrates how institutional and citizen efforts can combine to create expanded capacity and new forms of community engagement
Community Appreciation (Gui et al., 2022)	Recognition of local non-profit work and volunteer contributions	Design intervention and interview study	Additive (volunteer support) and transformative (community awareness)	Shows importance of visibility and acknowledgment in care work
Disaster Relief (Jo et al., 2023, 2021)	COVID-19 community response through mutual aid	Interview study	Additive (immediate relief) and transformative (social change)	Shows how crisis response transformed recipients into active care providers
Hobbyist Community (Knearem et al., 2019)	Knowledge sharing in beer brewing community	Participant observations and interview study	Additive (knowledge pooling) and transformative (collaborative learning)	Fluid transitions between teaching and learning roles enable reciprocal growth

design interventions, allowing us to understand both the lived experience of participants and the practical considerations for supporting care coproduction. While situated within a particular geographic and cultural context, these studies reveal how coproduction of care enhances well-being for all involved.

2.1 Coproducing Care Within Families

The family is a source of care in a variety of ways, including health (Stuifbergen et al., 2008; Sun, 2016). In most families, there is a desire to help each other and contribute to the whole family's common good (Sun, 2016). Yet, not all families are active in cultivating good health together due to a variety reasons, including changing of family roles and member's lack of interest in healthy behaviors.

In most family units, there is a strong social order and structure. In terms of generational order, parents are the main providers of care when their children are younger. However, this care dynamic reverses to an extent as parents age and receive care from their adult children. Previous reports (PRC, 2015) show that with the increase of the older adult population, many young adults are taking the lead role as caregivers and assuming responsibility for the care of their aging parents, for example with health care. The change of caregiver roles has implications on the family dynamic and reciprocity of care. When children are grown and able to make decisions on their own, elderly parents attempt to find a balance between showing care and prying for information. Similarly, as elderly parents grow older, the adult children's struggle is between staying independent and providing care for them.

2.1.1 Demands for Independence in Traditional Family Care Dynamics

To unpack the challenges related to family role change and providing care for health, we conducted a study which sought the perspectives of people filling the roles of elderly parents and adult children in a family dynamic (Binda et al., 2018). We held in-person, semi-structured, scenario-based, focus-group sessions with each generation group to understand individuals' current practices and learn their existing obstacles with respect to this topic.

We learned that adult children were interested in producing care but there was a problem with such care being accepted by their parents. Our data showed that elderly parents presented resistance in accepting their children's care actions because they want to be independent and not feel babysat by their children. For example, one young adult participant said that her mother would resist receiving her acts of care because of a rigid view that care flows from the mother and to the daughter in a mother-daughter relationship (Binda et al., 2018).

We also learned that there are conflicting ways of thinking about care responsibilities. While adult children participants asserted their independence and expressed feeling annoyed when their parents ask a lot of questions about their health, elderly parents try to strike a balance between showing care and prying for information when they want to know about their adult children's lifestyle, including health status. For instance, one young adult participant mentioned that she felt like she was being grilled when her mom asked for information about her and her children's healthy behaviors.

On the other hand, elderly parents explained how hard this situation was for them as a parent because it is hard to find a balance. One older participant said that she thinks her children see her attempts to showing care as prying, being too parental, and still trying to hover over them when they are adults (Binda et al., 2018). In other words, the need for a sense of independence is mutual.

2.1.1.1 Increasing Sense of Independence via Reciprocal Roles

Given this challenging situation, we see an opportunity to apply the coproduction concept to deal with family production of care, specifically on health. As mentioned, both adult children and elderly parents need to have a sense of independence while producing care. We learned elderly parent may resist receiving care from their adult children. Thus, we argue that it cannot be taken for granted that the parent will accept the care from their adult children. However, coproduction emerges when caring interactions are accepted. In this context, additive coproduction can be seen when elderly parents start to accept care, to be open to receive care from their adult children, which gives an opportunity for cooperation.

As mentioned, coproduction implies a reciprocal relationship between providers and recipients. So, if elderly parents show resistance to their children's advice about diet, maybe adult children could try to make receiving this type care service more pleasant in order to facilitate its acceptance. For example, while visiting their parents, adult children may initiate a care service related to healthy diet and nutrition by cooking a healthy meal, which could facilitate elderly parents to join and to be more active in accepting the care from their children.

Finally, we observed the conflicting ways of thinking about care responsibilities between elderly parents and adult children (Binda et al., 2018). Parents may feel like they are babysat by their children when their children try to show care. On the other side, adult children may feel that their parents are still trying to hover over them. We see here an opportunity for coproduction of care to emerge and transform these caring interactions. Since in this family dynamic, the family roles are being changed, coproduction can transform the way of thinking from both providers and receivers of care in a way that changes what people are doing regularly. The change on production of care could convert both parties into active participants of care provision, turning it into a reciprocal interaction, and producing synergy within all parties involved, that can be seen as transformative.

Thus, we argue that coproducing care in this context may happen when families shift roles and a way of thinking about providers and recipients, and its dynamic becomes satisfactory and equal. For example, instead of prying for information from adult children and passively receiving care, elderly parents may become active in the service of care, and initiate it by sharing their own information on their lifestyle, e.g., exercises practices. At the same time, adult children may show care by reciprocally sharing information about their own attempts to be healthy as well as messages of support and encouragement to their parents' practices. This shift in attitude transforms this family dynamic when compared to the original way of thinking about care responsibilities.

2.1.2 Conflicts in Health Beliefs Within Traditional Family Care

In another case study, we sought the perspectives of people filling the roles of elderly parents and adult children in a family dynamic via semi-structured, one-on-one interviews, which allowed us to take a guided conversational approach (Sandbulte et al., 2021). In this study, we learned that family support is valuable to encourage members to engage in healthy living practices. However, some members' lack of interest in healthy living impacts their family's collaboration on health. While some family members share the same values and standards in terms of healthy habits, others may have different standards when it comes to the definition and practice of health and well-being. Those members seemed satisfied with their own thoughts and beliefs and decided to stick with them, which might limit collaborative interactions within their family (Sandbulte et al., 2021).

For example, one young adult mentioned that she and her sister share similar goals and values in terms of healthy eating. Meanwhile, their mother has different opinions and standards for healthy eating, and sees her role as one of providing care through guidance of her daughters eating habits, not joining the daughters in working toward healthy diets. According to one of the young adult participants, she has tried to show care to her mother by writing a healthy diet plan for her. She said that her intention was to help her mother by providing information on a nutritious diet. Yet her mother's response was dismissive.

2.1.2.1 Resolving Conflicts via Inviting to Coproducing Care

Since families may have existing conflicts due to individual differences in health beliefs, we see an opportunity to apply the coproduction concept to address this situation. Coproducing care would impact the family dynamic by focusing on the synergies of recognizing the capacity of people who are different from us and leveraging insights from different individuals to promote cooperation on health. More specifically, the coproduction view would *transform* family interactions regarding members' goals and values for healthy living by moving members to acknowledge another person's values despite their differences.

In addition, the coproduction view would promote family collaboration by *bringing together* members who have distinguished ideas to equally contribute to the family's common good. For instance, in the family case presented earlier, instead of one family member writing a healthy diet plan and giving it to other members, the family member could invite other members who share (or do not share) similar beliefs on health to participate in the planning, giving the opportunity for all family members to add ideas and share their thoughts. By bringing members together to cooperate equally, the strategy of presenting the right way of eating healthy to the family would be associated with the synergistic effect of coproduction.

2.2 Coproducing Care Between New Parents

The transition to parenthood typically involves a lot of uncertainty and stress, particularly as roles shift and expand from being a couple to being parents. While there are diverse family structures, we focus on co-parenting dynamics among heterosexual, cisgender couples in developed Western countries, reflecting the scope of our participant sample in this case study. The delight associated with having a baby doesn't negate the fact that parents, especially women, often experience lower levels of marital satisfaction than couples who don't have children (Twenge et al., 2003). A significant number of parents reported depressive symptoms (Perren et al., 2005). Stressful family environments in infancy can have lasting effects on children, even if parents later restore their mental health and relationship harmony (Wakschlag & Hans, 1999).

Contemporary society is witnessing a change in gender roles regarding childcare, especially with fathers being more involved in parenting than they were in the past (McKellar et al., 2006). In the context of developed Western countries, fathers are perceived as co-parents, actively participating in the development of their children (Ramchandani et al., 2013). In this context, it's essential for parents to collaborate and effectively communicate to manage family responsibilities, including tasks like changing diapers, selecting childcare options, addressing both mental and physical fatigue, and maintaining their romantic relationship. If two parents fail to actively communicate, coordinate, understand, and support each other, the stress of parenting can become overwhelming and may lead to lasting harm to their marriage. In the worst cases, family separations or divorces can occur, with over one in five parents ending their marriage within four years of having a child (CowanHetherington, 2013).

2.2.1 Challenges in Task Distribution and Values in Recognizing Efforts

To understand the co-parenting challenges, we conducted a semi-structured interview study with first-time parents in heterosexual, cisgender couples raising a child under the age of three to investigate how partners collaborate, support, and relate to each other (Lin et al., 2024). We found that parents' attitudes toward co-parenting practices are positive. They were willing to commit to collaborating with their partners and trust them. Furthermore, parents bear the common notion that they should be role models for their children. For instance, a father shared with us that, after the birth of his child, he was making progress in communicating with his wife, which had been an issue between them for a long time.

However, parents encountered a few challenges when parenting together. First, we found that although both mothers and fathers wanted to support each other, some parents still expressed that they did not get enough support from their partners. The task distribution was less preferable or leaned toward one of the two parents, or parents could not actively provide proper support due to various reasons, such as parents not knowing how much to support their partner, a child treating a mother and a father differently, and the preference and benefits of childrearing tasks not fully understood.

On the other hand, we also found that when parents found their partners needed help, they were understanding and accommodated them, such as covering up the tasks that were left. Parents were even willing to do the work they did not feel comfortable doing to support their partners. Parents also emotionally supported their partners when they were distressed, validating their partner's feelings and comforting each other. Last but not least, parents supported their partners' self-esteem. Parents considered recognition of efforts and competency trust from their partners critical to parenting. When their partners recognized their efforts, their confidence in parenting increased. Showing appreciation could be done in various ways, such as with words of affirmation, while some parents were not used to such explicit action.

Here, we see an opportunity to apply *additive* coproduction, which facilitates parents to understand each other more and know when to support each other. For example, sharing physical information (e.g., sleep and level of fatigue) and mental load (e.g., stress) are likely to help. Also, we could foster a mutual understanding of preferences, abilities, and efforts so that parents are better aware of each other's needs and, thus, find it easier to support each other both physically and mentally. Furthermore, we consider this give-and-receive interaction a *transformative* coproduction as the relationship is strengthened. When parents support each other in childcare tasks, their partners feel cared for, trusted, and loved, and thus their bond becomes stronger.

2.2.2 Navigating Disagreements and Finding Common Goals

Besides parents supporting each other, we found that parents had difficulties reaching a consensus and that emotions can impede communication. Though both parents bear the notion that they want the best for their child and family, they might not share the same notion of what is best. Although they tried to be a role model for their child, they sometimes had unwanted emotional conversations and raised their voices, triggering negative emotions. Some of them found it challenging to communicate due to their partner's lack of effort to listen.

On the other hand, we found that parents used some strategies to help the communication process, such as speaking in non-judgmental ways or talking about concerns instead of hiding them. Similarly, parents use various ways to find common ground. For example, one parent said that laying out each other's priorities after having a child helps them learn the determination of their partner to work on a difficult shared task. One common family goal parents mentioned was to be positive role models for their children.

Their strategies reflect Carroll et al. (2016), which sees parties in coproduction as initiators and joiners; initiators suggest an action, and the joiners agree or provide modified actions; then both parties conduct the action together and recognize each other's efforts for working on their actions. For example, parents agreed and tried to handle disagreements more amicably in front of their children, such as by avoiding conflicts or having respectful debates that could serve as a learning opportunity for their children. When one parent initiated good role model behavior, another joined and behaved similarly. Both parents designed and criticized their own modeling and their partner's modeling, then executed agreed-upon parenting together. Furthermore, as a family, parents respect each family member's individual and common goals. A parent even visualized these goals to remind them of being a family. These actions can improve both the couple's relationship and the well-being of their child. We considered these efforts as a process towards *transformative* coproduction as parents became better at communicating with their partners afterward. Also, two parents can have both of their voices heard and be concerned.

2.3 People with Different Abilities Coproducing Care Through Collaborative Shopping

The term *people with visual impairment* (PVI) normally refers to people with vision loss or people who have visual impairment even with corrective devices (e.g., glasses). This group may seem vulnerable to sighted people and can be considered as marginalized in Cahn's view of community-supported care provision. In this case study, we investigated collaborative shopping practices between PVI and their sighted family members or friends, in which the PVI is not only receiving caring assistance, but actively contributing to the shopping task through equal participation.

When shopping together, it is a common practice that the sighted people provide physical guidance to the PVI by offering their elbows. This allows PVI to grasp their arms slightly above the elbows and follow their movements easily. In this collaborative activity, the sighted people are in control of the navigation, while PVI could cooperate in the physical movements and at the same time generate confirmation and clarification on the items they intend to buy. They are caring one another by noticing and accommodating each other's needs. We see this collaborative shopping practice from a more additive perspective of coproduced care, because they have predefined roles and are adding strengths together to complete the shopping tasks. However, in some scenarios where PVI play a more active role, we show how a transformative care is incidentally produced from such routine practice.

2.3.1 Recognizing Capabilities for Transformative Coproduction

In our case study of how PVI use a commercially available remote assistive service (Lee et al., 2020), we learned that PVI still tend to use assistive technologies even if their sighted family members are nearby. For instance, when a husband and wife were shopping together, the husband (our participant), who experiences blindness, called for a live agent and asked for remote sighted assistance even though he was shopping with his sighted wife. They were sharing a shopping list and getting the items separately, which made the shopping trip more efficient. Our participant asked the remote agent to navigate and to read the text on packages for him so that he could make a choice on which items to buy. If he could not decide, he would take the items to his wife and discuss them and they would make the final decision together.

In this shopping interaction, our participant was not waiting for his wife to get all of the items on their list, but trying to provide help and give care to her. Although getting each item was more challenging for him, he knew he could bring items he was unsure about to his wife to ask for her opinion, and they could decide together whether or not to purchase it. The husband showed respect to his wife. This couple's shopping practice can be seen from a transformative coproduction lens, where the emphasis is put on what people can do rather than what they cannot do (Glynos & Speed, 2012). The participant who experiences blindness is not only a care recipient but also a care producer. Although his visual impairment impedes his free movement through the store, he gives care to his wife by actively helping with the shopping trip, even though he requires remote sighted assistance. He also offers emotional support to his wife through communicating with her, making her feel a sense of comfort and being respected.

In another example of a couple shopping together, a partially sighted female participant shared a story about a recent shopping trip with her sighted husband, which showcased how their individual strengths contributed to reciprocal care production. When grocery shopping, our participant usually took charge because she is better at planning the grocery list than her husband. Normally her husband drives her to the location and waits in the parking lot, while she goes inside the store and gets all their groceries. She is familiar with the layout and can communicate with the shop assistants well, therefore, most of the time she can efficiently complete the shopping task alone even though she has a visual impairment. On the other hand, when they are shopping at a home repair store, a "men's store", like Home Depot, she will push the cart a little slower behind her husband because she is not familiar with the route. She enjoys learning the new vocabulary of all kinds of tools from her husband during the shopping. The husband is good at driving and calculating the price, while the wife is better at remembering the route and communicating with people in the stores.

A synergy is generated from their mutual recognizing capabilities. In their shopping practice, both of them enjoy the activities and appreciate the contributions of each other, which illustrates mutual caring. The partially sighted participant said she never felt babied by her husband, and received direct help only when she asked for it. She sees her husband's patiently waiting in the parking lot while she shops inside as a respectful gesture. The care they coproduced in these shopping activities carries a transformative accent because their roles are not pre-defined (Glynos & Speed, 2012). Either of them could be the initiator of a shopping trip, and they take roles initiating and joining according to their strengths while also supporting one another. In this way, the reciprocity of mutual care may arise.

2.4 Coproducing Care and Environmental Health Through Community-Based Monitoring

Threat to environmental resources and climate change is one of the biggest global concerns. Even though government agencies and professional scientists have had an institutional role in dealing with this crisis, lack of resources and socio-political turmoil have rendered their efforts inadequate (Agrawal & Gibson, 1999). This has forced institutions to reconsider the role of citizens in natural resource management and decision-making. Community-based monitoring is the practice of citizens, government, academia, and other community institutions working together towards a local environmental issue (Conrad & Hilchey, 2011). Community-based monitoring is a broader term used to describe any kind of citizen-based environmental monitoring and management activity.

Citizen science is a community-based monitoring approach, where citizens participate in scientific endeavors in different ways (Little et al., 2016). Citizens may participate as volunteers assisting scientists in activities such as data collection, transcription, categorization, and analysis, or may work as part of a community hobby group, enthusiastic about conserving their natural resources and environment (Bonney et al., 2014). Citizen science, is hence a community of practice (Wenger, 2011) that promotes social benefit and strengthens communities by creating an environment of informal learning, community engagement, and awareness about local issues (Carroll et al., 2018).

We worked with community-based water monitoring groups in the Spring Creek Watershed to understand how this community of practice aids coproduction of care and better health by working towards safeguarding community water. Water quality monitoring and management is an important environmental domain where community-based monitoring activity has shown a positive correlation with a stronger watershed system (Grant & Langpap, 2019). Today, there are thousands of community-based water monitoring groups across the United States (ACWI, 2024). Although water quality monitoring has traditionally been a government enterprise, citizen groups both change and add to that capacity.

We identified 13 community-based water monitoring groups that consisted of citizens, government officials, non-profits, and academics, collaboratively working together. We conducted interviews, workshops, and field observations to understand their practices. The interviews and field observations helped us understand the individual socio-technical practices, and the workshops helped us understand how this community of practice as a whole coproduced environmental health and care for the community.

2.4.1 Additive and Transformative Citizen Science

The practice of citizen science has especially proliferated and gained traction in environmental science where researchers need to collect large volumes of data over a wide geographical area (Silvertown, 2009). In environmental sciences, there has been a long history of citizens collecting and recording observations to help them understand the natural world.

With professionalization of science, the knowledge of these 'amateur' citizens got excluded (Cornwell & Campbell, 2012). Collaboration between citizens and scientists allows citizens to share and add their knowledge to institutional science. Hence, citizen science leads to not just coproduction of scientific knowledge, but also better environmental health.

In most citizen science projects, scientists are initiators of the coproduction activity and citizens are joiners. Such coproduction can be both additive and transformative. It is additive because citizens participating as data collectors add to the capacity of scientific work. Whereas, citizen science groups that are more autonomous and do not directly work under the guidance of a professional scientist or organization are transforming their community's environmental resources. On the other hand, extreme citizen science (Stevens et al., 2014) is a transformative movement, as it involves participation of marginalized communities aimed towards social and political change in third-world communities.

2.4.2 Hackathon to Share Stakes and Transform Roles of Stakeholders

We conducted hackathon style workshops that created an agile environment to discuss and come up with design solutions and challenges. The implication of these sessions was not just creation of design scenarios but also creation of a unique synergy through discussions in a highly motivated and active community. Participants considered the design hackathons to be events that brought all water stakeholders and residents together and facilitated exchange of information and ideas. In addition, the healthy and constructive discussion during each event led participants to critically assess and analyze scenarios.

This event was an example of transformative coproduction because it created an environment of mutual learning and brought people together in a participatory design context. It brought together various water stakeholders (residents and water monitoring groups) to share problems in their water system, discuss the kind of tools needed to address these problems, and why they would want those tools. It also led to a role change, where everybody was now playing a new role as a designer (facilitated by us), and the residents were becoming a part of the discussion about tools for water monitoring which is a rather invisible and arcane activity that's going on in the community, but is none the less important. People were contributing not just according to their role but according to roles that are surprising that they usually don't take on. It transformed the way water stakeholders contemplated their water system and their community. It led them to talk about the future, in terms of design and tools that none of them had actually used but some of them might use in the future.

2.4.3 Citizen-Based Water Monitoring Increasing Synergies in Local Communities

Learning about individual groups helped us understand how their practices added to the capacity of scientific and civic endeavors. The large population of older adults in this community was a driver and a fruitful element for citizen-based monitoring activity. For instance, Pennsylvania Senior Environmental Corps (PaSEC) is a non-profit volunteer organization of older adults who monitor streams in Spring Creek Watershed. They collect baseline water quality data that can be used for trend analysis, decision-making, and educating the community about their water system. PaSEC's monitoring activities complement civic conservation initiatives by providing additional data, thereby providing resources for better water quality to the community. Moreover, the monitoring activity itself is a healthy venture for the participating older adults. Water quality monitoring is a strenuous physical activity that provides significant physical exercise, and builds social capital that nurtures participants' mental health and well-being. In addition to adding to the civic water monitoring efforts, PaSEC also takes initiatives to engage with the broader community by creating programs to involve school kids in monitoring activities.

Similarly, the Spring Creek Chapter of Trout Unlimited is another non-profit volunteer organization that aims to conserve and restore cold-water fisheries. It has active volunteers who often work as citizen scientists for researchers at Penn State. Having a large network of volunteers to gather data for a scientific project helps researchers cover wider geographic area for a relatively small cost. At the same time, these volunteers also engage in other conservation and water management activities such as building riparian buffers to protect stormwater runoff.

Besides implicitly adding to institutional efforts, we found instances where citizen-based monitoring was directly augmenting community's water system. The Water Resources Monitoring Program (WRMP) is a committee formed by citizen-based groups in the Spring Creek Watershed, to collect and maintain a repository of baseline water quality data. This data is often used by local Borough Water Authority and Sewer Authority, to meet regulatory compliance. It is also used by both citizen and government water groups to compare and predict trends in water quality over time.

The efforts of the community-based water monitoring groups in the Spring Creek Watershed do more than just safeguard local water system. The water monitoring activity brings the community together to share, learn and teach each other about their environment. The citizen scientists participate in these activities because they care about their community and hence are implicitly motivated to work towards ensuring safe water for the community. Hence, community-based monitoring groups coproduce scientific knowledge, environmental health and care for their community. Hence, such transformative and additive coproduction not just add to civic and scientific efforts, but also creates synergy in the community.

2.5 Coproducing Care Through Community Appreciation

Non-profit groups have been supporting local communities by strengthening their ability to grow and caring for the ones in need. Local volunteers are local community members. They serve the communities they live in and work on issues that closely impact the neighbors' lives. Prior research has found that receiving acknowledgment helps to sustain volunteer activity (Fisher & Ackerman, 1998; Tan et al., 2020; Winterich et al., 2013), but the impact of acknowledgment can be more substantial. In this section, we discuss coproducing care through community acknowledgment, and how it can enable both additive and transformative coproduction. Community care can be coproduced additively when acknowledgment is from people who are already aware of the non-profits. It can also be transformatively coproduced through facilitating acknowledgment from people who are unfamiliar with local non-profits' work. We present a case study illustrating both types of coproduction.

2.5.1 Lack of Visibility to Local Non-profit Groups

Many non-profits groups in the local community take action to care for people in need. These groups provide services for a variety of needs including food insecurity, firefighting, animal care, and environmental issues. Specifically in State College, PA, State College Meals on Wheels volunteers dedicated their time to deliver food to homebound residents, the Alpha Fire Company firefighters step in during emergency fire situations, and senior citizen volunteers in PaSEC (see Sect. 3.3) test and monitor the water quality of local streams.

The care these groups provide is crucial and can be beneficial to anyone in the local community. However, many of their efforts are not visible. Local community members who have lived in the community for a long time are often unaware of many of these groups. On the other side, some non-profit groups also recognize a lack of visibility in the local community, and they seek ways to improve. For community members who are aware of these services, they might appreciate volunteers' work, but do not have a platform that motivates them to share their awareness or acknowledgment. Facilitating community acknowledgment could be one approach to increase the groups' visibility and improve volunteer experiences.

2.5.2 Thank-You Station for Coproducing Care Between Volunteers and Local Members

To understand how community acknowledgment influences the experiences of volunteers and community members, we set up two thank-you stations in public locations in the local community to invite community members to write a thank-you card to local non-profit groups. Thank you cards might be familiar to volunteer groups, however, it is often from the ones who are well aware of the volunteer services or who have received services from them. Through our thank-you stations, we explored how local volunteers respond to acknowledgment from unfamiliar community members. After collecting thank you cards from the stations, we conducted semi-structured interviews with five volunteers involved in local volunteer groups, and three community members who participated in thank you card writing and viewing. Each interview lasted from 15 to 30 min, and all interviews were audio-recorded and transcribed. We then conducted a thematic analysis of the interview data. For additional information, please see Gui et al. (2022).

Previous studies showed that acknowledgment could help volunteers to sustain their work and increase volunteer engagement (Fisher & Ackerman, 1998; Tan et al., 2020; Winterich et al., 2013). We also found that volunteers enjoyed different forms of acknowledgment, including the acknowledgment from their managers, donors, or previously served community members. The acknowledgment from those who are familiar to the volunteers is an example of additive coproduction. The acknowledgments confirmed the value of these volunteer services and encouraged volunteers to sustain their contribution to the local community. In this case, people who gave acknowledgment were the initiators in this coproduction process as they took time and effort to praise volunteers' hard work. This action urged volunteers as joiners to continue their contribution to the community, thus they came together to produce more care in the community.

Besides the additive coproduction example, we also identified a transformative coproduction process through the acknowledgment activity at our thank-you stations, especially when thank-you card writers were previously unfamiliar to the volunteer groups. It was transformative because the roles of caregivers and care receivers changed several times during this process. The coproduction process started with volunteers dedicating their time to care for their local community. They tested the water quality, rescued injured animals, provided free medical care, and delivered many other forms of care to the local community. These activities benefited anyone who lives in the local community, thus volunteers served as initiators while community members were care receivers. Through the thank you card writing activity, community members who were originally care receivers then had the chance to care for the volunteers by acknowledging their work. Local community members' role of care receivers changed into joiners. In this process, local community members who were previously unfamiliar to the volunteer group also became aware of the group. This change made volunteers' work more visible, to experience the joy of being appreciated, and to gain the assurance of their work quality.

Moreover, as the community members became familiar with more local volunteer groups, they also received awareness of care. It allowed the community members to learn about the local community resources for future needs and to build confidence in the local community's collective efficacy. Besides these direct effects from the thank you note stations, indirect effects also exist to benefit the local community. Volunteers are more likely to sustain their work as volunteers when their work is recognized, thus they would be more likely to continue to take actions to care for the local community. Community members who did not participate in the thank you note writing can also benefit from such an activity.

2.6 Coproducing Community Care and Resilience Towards Prolonging Crises

Demands for various forms of care and populations requiring care increase and diversify when disasters strike. Such phenomena were prominent during COVID-19, which the World Health Organization declared a global pandemic on March 11, 2020 (WHO, 2020) and prolonged for over two years. With the pandemic damaging numerous geographic communities simultaneously, governments worldwide imposed interventions that undermined human connections to prevent the spread of the virus, including shelter-in-place orders and restrictions on social gatherings. As a result, economic and social damages were incurred, as well as healthcare crises. Immunocompromised individuals did not feel safe leaving their houses, there were shortages in personal protective equipment (PPE), and healthcare providers suffered from a surge in workloads. Severe economic damages and subsequent high-rocketing layoffs aggravated and brought food and housing insecurity to the surface. With physical distancing measures driving social interaction online, information and communication technologies (ICT) became more vital than ever to enable ordinary life activity, exacerbating the digital divide. Those not equipped with digital devices or internet connections were inadvertently excluded from participating fully in work or learning.

Government resources stretched thin to meet increasing and diverse needs, and we found that citizens voluntarily stepped in to fill the gaps in care by supporting each other during the pandemic. To understand the generic coordination process and impacts of multiple initiatives, we conducted an interview study with 17 civic initiative volunteers in the United States who participated in bottom-up, citizen-driven disaster relief activities.

In addition, we took notice of the person-to-person online mutual aid which bloomed across the United States in the early days of the pandemic. In online mutual aid groups, members exchange information, ask for various kinds of help, and offer to provide help for others. Participation is open to anyone in the community. We conducted an analysis of the most utilized mutual aid platforms and conducted interviews with 17 mutual aid group administrators.

Community fridge groups were another social movement that grew in response to the pandemic. Following the pandemic, economic crises brought food insecurity to the forefront. Locals placed refrigerators in publicly accessible areas to feed neighbors and reduce food waste. We interviewed 17 community fridge group members from across the United States to understand their core values and impacts, as well as how they dealt with any challenges they encountered.

In this section, we illustrate how these citizen-led movements enacted additive and transformative care to alleviate the prolonging crises of the pandemic and food insecurity, and discuss the considerations and benefits of coproducing care that emerged from our case studies.

2.6.1 Additive Coproduction of Disaster Relief: Filling in the Gaps in Formal Disaster Response

From a broad perspective, these civic initiatives were an additive coproduction of disaster relief. Those with distinct resources and skills formed a local expert network and complemented disaster relief from government and formal agencies, serving as "double capacities." They ensured that local hospitals did not run out of PPE, fed food-insecure individuals, and expressed gratitude to encourage overburdened frontline workers. These civic initiatives were viable because each individual creatively adapted and mobilized their available resources or abilities, rather than making contributions in unfamiliar ways (Jo et al., 2021). Local distilleries shifted their focus to produce hand sanitizer, while a family-run business for making snow skis manufactured plastic face shields. A college faculty in the Department of Mechanical Engineering and the local maker space collaborated to 3D print face shields; school athletic uniform makers and local independent theaters collaborated to create a digital pattern for gowns and sew gowns and masks; and faculty in the College of Business managed supply chain systems to efficiently distribute fabricated PPE to local hospitals and nursing homes. Fitness professionals, comedians, and tattoo artists raised fundraising events, and individuals purchased meals from local restaurants, financially struggling due to no-dining-in measures, who cooked and delivered meals to food insecure individuals and frontline workers with a thank-you letter. People donated laptops or other computer accessories no longer in use; retired programmers wiped out data from them; and local non-profit organizations connected them to students in need of digital devices, due to most schools moving to online learning. More details can be found in Jo et al. (2021).

Similar to civic initiatives, mutual aid groups were a source of support for people who were adversely affected by the virus or pandemic-related disruptions to daily life, in tandem with governmental efforts. For example, food was a frequently requested item in almost all of the groups we examined. Many mutual aid participants contributed towards immediate food relief for their neighbors via cash donations to individuals, grocery delivery and community-organized meals (Knearem et al., 2021). These actions reduced hunger in the community as a form of care through *food dignity*, emphasizing that all people should have a choice in what they eat.

2.6.2 Transformative Coproduction of Disaster Relief: Citizens and Marginalized Populations as Support Providers

Participation in coproducing disaster relief transformed the role of citizens, who are frequently viewed as recipients of formal aid. For instance, they actively assisted frontline workers, who usually do not receive support under the traditional disaster relief model, ensuring that local hospitals and nursing homes did not run out of PPE and appreciating and encouraging frontline workers overburdened for an extended period of the pandemic. Citizens also benefited from coproducing disaster relief. Many of our participants stated that they felt helpless and bad for those working on the frontlines prior to joining coproducing relief. As they coproduced care for one another, they felt psychologically rewarded for making tangible social impacts rather than passively receiving aid, which resulted in an increased sense of hope amidst the pandemic (Jo et al., 2023).

We also identified transformative changes in the roles of initiators and joiners. Frontline workers initiated disaster relief, and citizens joined by donating money to purchase hot meals for them, and local restaurants joined by offering discounts and delivering meals with thank-you letters. Throughout this citizen-led activity, others joined and initiated fundraising events. When healthcare workers received meals, they joined the support network by ordering from the local restaurants in return for financial support. The chain of initiators and joiners helped the local community holistically survive the long-haul crises.

Mutual aid favors a non-hierarchical organizational structure, which lends itself towards transformative care. We found that mutual aid members took fluid roles in the group, as aid requesters (e.g., asking their neighbors for specific support) or aid providers (e.g., fulfilling someone else's request), depending on their situation at the time (Knearem et al., 2021). Each person could take multiple roles in the group simultaneously or by switching between them; for example by requesting one type of aid, while also being able to offer a different type of aid to fulfill someone else's request.

Community fridges also showed the vivid advantages of transforming care activities and engaging those who are often marginalized. The management of community fridges involved individuals who benefited from government food assistance and were often viewed as passive care recipients. They had firsthand experience with the shortfalls of traditional custodial care, which followed formalized systems for efficiency, requesting applications, operating within fixed hours at limited locations, or offering a limited option of fresh food. They understood how formal custodial care could inadvertently induce feelings of shame and self-stigma of being "needy" when visiting food banks or having prearranged food boxes handed over from authorities behind a table.

By taking part in the management of community fridges, these individuals gained agency over their care and incorporated their values and perspectives. A fundamental principle of community fridges was that they were 24/7 open to anyone, regardless of whether they were food insecure or not, allowing individuals to choose what food to take without the presence or judgement of others, removing the stigma attached to getting free food. Volunteers made decisions about the use of donations, the placement of new community fridges, and when and how they wanted to volunteer. Individuals took food from community fridges and offered what they could, whether it be food, money, time, or labor, without feeling indebted or ashamed. In this manner, those typically seen merely as care recipients also became care providers, offering valuable insights to effectively provide food assistance or contributing to the maintenance of fridges or the construction of fridge shelters.

2.6.3 Care Cannot be Automatically Delivered

We also witnessed unintended consequences in less transformative coproduction from another citizen-led disaster relief activity distributing donated laptops to students. As knowledge cannot be simply "delivered" to those in need unless they are willing to learn, volunteers had some students refuse to receive donated laptops, although they explained that they were free of cost (Jo et al., 2023). Volunteers did not understand the reasons behind their refusals, and their endeavors to provide disaster relief occasionally did not move forward. While engaging all relevant stakeholders is a key to transformative coproduction, in reality, it is easier to involve people who share similar backgrounds than to engage those who are less alike. Individuals on the wrong side of the digital divide might not fully recognize the benefits of technology, and misconceptions about technology could have led to their refusal.

As we have seen in the community fridge example, care could have been more successfully delivered if relief activity had been more transformatively conceptualized, for example, if those with more limited access to information technology had been regarded as assets to volunteers trying to address the full range of care provision. This example demonstrates that care might not always be accepted when the reciprocal participation of care recipients is not engaged in its production and delivery.

2.6.4 Benefits of Coproducing Disaster Relief: Increased Collective Resilience and the Role of Visibility

Broadly speaking, the production of disaster relief manifested as community care, i.e., showing appreciation for helpers in the community, supporting one another's physical, emotional and mental health needs needs and engaging in fulfilling social interactions online, all of which can bring visibility to community beliefs (i.e., community-collective efficacy) and capacities (i.e., resilience) (Knearem et al., 2022). Coproducing disaster relief gradually increased collective efficacy, an individual's *belief* in their community's capacity to overcome challenges, leading to collective resilience, the *product* of realized collective efforts that enables recovery from collective adversity (Goddard et al., 2004). Before COVID-19, people knew that vulnerable members always existed, but they did not take the issue seriously enough to take action or were unsure of where to start. The outbreak of COVID-19 arranged a social capital network of coproducing care and enhanced individuals' belief in what they are capable of toward others in their local communities (Jo et al., 2023). One of the relief groups initially aimed to provide meals to healthcare workers and support local businesses, but throughout the pandemic, they noticed the worsening conditions of marginalized populations already struggling with food and housing insecurity pre-pandemic. Consequently, the group broadened their relief efforts to include these populations as well and aspired to continue caring for neighbors even after the pandemic.

We noticed that making impacts of group performance visible was vital in further enhancing collective efficacy and resilience (Jo et al., 2021). Several relief groups updated the number of populations who benefited from their efforts to publicize successful group performance and attract more people to join their cause. In terms of community fridges, prior to their physical installation in a neighborhood, many locals were skeptical about their feasibility and sustainability. However, once a community fridge was placed on a sidewalk, stocked with surplus food, and fed people, they saw its immediate benefits to the community and were convinced of its effective operation. This increased sense of collective efficacy motivated more local members to join in using and managing community fridges. These joiners initiated other relief efforts, building dry shelves next to fridges to share items like clothing, feminine hygiene products, baby essentials, first aid kits, and facial masks, or organizing clothing or school supply drives. One of our participants noted that the community fridge was a starting point for the community to organize support networks.

In a second example, online group members brought awareness to other's good deeds and elevated pro-social initiatives. We observed people appreciating both frontline healthcare workers as well as a wider range of community members including mask makers, food donors and people who provided goods to families in need. The roles being appreciated in the group were not commonly considered during the pandemic, as most acts of appreciation that made the national news were directed to frontline workers terms of showing appreciation (Webber et al., 2020). For instance, the collective gratitude shown towards mask makers early in the pandemic shed visibility on a previously unrecognized community asset; this particular asset is vital to effective disaster relief during a long-haul disaster. The posts of appreciation in the online group helped group members become aware of individual mask makers contributions, which can increase member's beliefs that their community can cope with a difficult situation together where there was a dearth of PPE early on in the pandemic (Knearem et al., 2022).

In yet another example, increased visibility led not only to more local individuals joining relief efforts but also to people in other communities starting similar initiatives. Our participants shared that they were inspired by relief efforts they learned about online and were motivated by the potential impact they could make. Conversely, two participants detailed their strategies for supporting local communities online, including instructional guides to encourage replication of their initiatives. This prompted individuals from various communities to seek advice and initiate similar projects in their own areas. One participant recounted discovering open-source 3D-printed designs for plastic face shields shared by a research institute abroad. He modified these designs to enhance durability and reduce production time to support his local hospitals, initiating relief efforts to manufacture PPE. By sharing these improved designs online, he also joined a broader network of care, extending support across different communities and even internationally.

2.6.5 Benefits of Transformative Disaster Relief: Collective Actualization

In the mutual aid example, similarities in forms of care emerged across the groups that we examined, which suggests that even though the specific type of need and intensity of need may vary by group, all of the groups went through similar evolutionary phases as facilitators of disaster relief. From this work, we proposed the mutual aid hierarchy of community needs (Knearem et al., 2024), based on Maslow's hierarchy of needs (McLeod, 2007). The hierarchy comprises of identifying and addressing immediate needs at the bottom layer, then developing long-term support for chronic needs in the middle layer, with transforming social systems comprising the upper-most layer. This represents a shift towards less concrete and more ambitious systemic and symbolic goals. Once online mutual aid groups were able to satisfy lower level needs, i.e., immediate and chronic needs, members began to think about their responsibility towards their community and the others living in it in a more abstract way. This kind of thinking represents a fundamental shift from concrete disaster relief to actualizing one's vision of their ideal community.

Thinking about the local community as an abstract system represents a higher order of thinking than the level of reflection required to react to one's own individual challenges. By reacting to the system, people are able to collectively consider what their ideals of social justice may look like and how they can get from where they are to where they would ideally like their society to be. Such initiatives born of collective reckoning with social justice can hold massive impact on local communities, regardless of whether or not they are the "right" or proper solution to the problem for the local community. What matters most at the upper-most layer is not whether the social justice initiatives that were brought up or organized through mutual aid groups are the *right* solutions for the local community; rather it matters that people have arrived at this level of thinking and believe that themselves and others should be thinking about and searching for answers to chronic community problems. It represents collective actualization, whereby the community, being satisfied in their basic needs, can now find motivation in other higher ways, striving for potential beyond what is currently imaginable (Maslow, 1967).

2.7 Sharing Knowledge as a Form of Care in a Hobbyist Community

Coproduction occurs when two or more parties actively pursue activities together that are reciprocal in nature (Cahn, 2010; Ostrom, 1996), with an emphasis on collaborative participation and role equality (Brandsen & Honingh, 2016). Sharing knowledge is a form of care that is coproduced both as additive through the traditional teacher/learner model and transformative when parties blur the lines between the teacher and learner role through collaborative learning. In the following case study, we discuss the coproduction of care through the lens of creativity support within a hobby beer-making community. Specifically, we investigated the practices around sharing knowledge as a form of care in beer-making (Knearem et al., 2019).

Brewing beer as a hobby is a popular activity in the United States, with approximately 1.1 million people engaged in the craft in 2017, 40% of whom began brewing four or less years prior (Brewers Association, 2017). Home brewers can be found across the United States and make a variety of beer styles. The home brewing community is a vast network of practitioners who are connected to each other through their shared interest in making their own beer. Home brewing clubs are prevalent in many locations across the United States and can be categorized as inviting and encouraging of people of all skill and interest levels to join.

We investigated a local home brew club located in the East Coast of the United States, which was representative of clubs located in similarly populated areas. Members range in experience level from beer enthusiasts who are curious about home brewing to professional brewers. Members are enthusiastic in offering advice, expertise or tools to support their fellow home brewers to create better beer. After building a relationship with the members of the home brewing community, we conducted interviews and participant observations.

We interviewed 11 home brewers, nine of which were members of a home brewing club. The other two members were recruited via snowball sampling and were newcomers to the craft who did not belong to a home brew club. The semi-structured interviews lasted between 60 minutes and 90 minutes. Among the interviewees, 10 were male and one was female. They had a wide variety of brewing experience ranging from less than a year to more than 30 years. Second, we conducted participant observations sessions where we engaged with club members as they participated in club activities (e.g collaborative brew days, club meetings, and beer festivals). All participants gave consent to be included in the study. See Knearem et al. (2019) for additional information.

2.7.1 Initiating and Joining Beer Brewing Activities

We found that care within the home brewing community was demonstrated through a variety of resource sharing activities (e.g., sharing knowledge about the craft, lending/borrowing materials and tools, and offering up one's own hobby space to others). Brewing handcrafted beer is often a solitary activity, however the frequency of engagement in such communal activities suggests that members gain more than the mere completion of their task or goal, rather they experience gains in both expertise and social support that are necessary to become more skillful brewers. In this section, we use the example of knowledge sharing to illustrate how care can be coproduced both additively and transformationally in the home brewing community.

Our participants frequently shared knowledge with each other during in-person home brew club activities. In this first example, a club member (i.e., the initiator) offers to teach other home brewers about an aspect of home brewing that they are knowledgeable in. Joiners are the other club members who actively engage in learning by participating in the initiator's activity. During a club meeting participant observation, we observed a blind beer tasting activity. The initiator organized the activity and began by pouring samples of beer for the members to taste. He then guided them through a beer tasting exercise where they learned how various ingredients contributed to each beer's flavor and appearance. Club members took notes on the worksheet provided for the activity. The initiator's role was to convey knowledge through a hands-on activity, which supported the joiners to *actively* engage in their own education. In this teacher/learner model, the initiator took a role of teacher, while the club members, i.e., joiners, assumed roles as students, actively participating in their own education. Learning how various ingredients worked together provided the opportunity for club members to apply this new knowledge to their brewing, and gave them ideas for future recipes, demonstrating how care within the brewing community can lead to positive outcomes for the individual home brewer's products.

In a second example, a club member described to others how he handled a problem with an off-flavor taste in his beer. He couldn't figure out what he did wrong so he brought his off-flavor beer to the home brew club meeting to ask the other brewers for advice. They tasted the beer and gave him feedback based on their brewing knowledge or past experience. One suggested more thorough equipment cleaning while another chemistry-oriented member pointed to a chemical compound that could have produced the undesirable flavor. The club member who initiated the discussion did not know about the chemical compound, and was able to understand from the others how to avoid it in the future. This example illustrates the fluid roles in a coproduction dynamic, i.e., once the conversation was initiated, the other brewers (as joiners) shifted between knowledge providers and consumers. The chemistry-oriented brewer's role shifted from a that of a joiner to an initiator when he shared his knowledge of chemistry with the group, and was asked to explain in detail. The other brewers (including our participant) took the role of joiners who actively took part in the conversation and learned something new from this spontaneous interaction. The result of this example was not only that the club member with the off-flavor beer was able to understand what happened to his beer, but that the entire group gained knowledge as a benefit of engaging in the conversation.

In a third example, participants told us that they engaged in collaborative brewing activities with other members of the home brewing club. We were invited to observe one such occurrence where a professional brewer at a local microbrewery offered up his brewery's equipment so that members of the club could come together to make a large batch of one of their recipes. The professional brewer initiated the activity by offering his location and brewing equipment, and the joiners were the members of the club who participated in the collaborative brew. The initiator procured the ingredients needed for a large batch based on the original recipe that the home brewers provided. At the beginning, he gave a short tutorial on how brewing on large equipment differs from home brewing. After this, they all went to work to make the beer. We observed as the group interacted and noticed that both parties were learning things from each other, building their expertise and complementing each other's skills while simultaneously coming together as a coherent group to reach their goal. The home brewers took turns reading out the instructions, adding ingredients, stirring the mixture, tasting at certain intervals, and taking notes on the process. The professional brewer would sometimes step in to demonstrate how to perform tasks, but left it to each individual to decide if and how they wanted to participate.

Here, the teacher/learner model that we noticed in the first and second example was transformed, as the line between providing and receiving information blurred. What emerged was collaborative learning; i.e., each participant was on equal standing in relation to the others, with significance placed on doing and discovering things together. Sharing knowledge through collectively engaging in an activity of mutual interest supported all the brewers to achieve their goal of making a large batch of beer on a professional scale. Each participant deepened their brewing skills via discussions and observing each other, strengthening their collective identity as beer brewers. While in the end they created a satisfying product, on top of that they collectively gained a new experience and increased social support, which can advance and deepen trust and belonging in home brewing community.

References

Advisory Committee on Water Information. (2024). Monitoring. Retrieved March 17, 2024.

Agrawal, A., & Gibson, C. C. (1999). Enchantment and disenchantment: The role of community in natural resource conservation. *World Development, 27*(4), 629–649.

Binda, J., Yuan, C. W., Cope, N., Park, H., Choe, E. K., & Carroll, J. M. (2018). Supporting effective sharing of health information among intergenerational family members. In *Proceedings of the 12th EAI International Conference on Pervasive Computing Technologies for Healthcare* (pp. 48–157).

Bonney, R., Shirk, J. L., Phillips, T. B., Wiggins, A., Ballard, H. L., Miller-Rushing, A. J., & Parrish, J. K. (2014). Next steps for citizen science. *Science, 343*(6178), 1436–1437.

Brandsen, T., & Honingh, M. (2016). Distinguishing different types of coproduction: A conceptual analysis based on the classical definitions. *Public Administration Review, 76*(3), 427–435.

Brewers Association. (2017). Study: 1.1 million Americans homebrew beer. Retrieved March 17, 2024, from https://www.brewersassociation.org/press-releases/study-1-1-million-americans-homebrew-beer/

Cahn, E. (2010). Co-production 2.0: Retrofitting human service programs to tap the renewable energy of community. *Community Currency Magazine, 8*, 36–39.

Carroll, J. M., Beck, J., Dhanorkar, S., Binda, J., Gupta, S., & Zhu, H. (2018). Strengthening community data: Towards pervasive participation. In *Proceedings of the 19th Annual International Conference on Digital Government Research: Governance in the Data Age* (pp. 1–9).

Carroll, J. M., Chen, J., Yuan, C. W. T., & Hanrahan, B. V. (2016). In search of coproduction: Smart services as reciprocal activities. *Computer, 49*(7), 26–32.

Conrad, C. C., & Hilchey, K. G. (2011). A review of citizen science and community-based environmental monitoring: Issues and opportunities. *Environmental Monitoring and Assessment, 176*, 273–291.

Cornwell, M. L., & Campbell, L. M. (2012). Co-producing conservation and knowledge: Citizen-based sea turtle monitoring in North Carolina, USA. *Social Studies of Science, 42*(1), 101–120.

Cowan, P. A., & Hetherington, E. M. (2013). *Family transitions*. Routledge.

Fisher, R. J., & Ackerman, D. (1998). The effects of recognition and group need on volunteerism: A social norm perspective. *Journal of Consumer Research, 25*(3), 262–275.

Glynos, J., & Speed, E. (2012). Varieties of co-production in public services: Time banks in a UK health policy context. *Critical Policy Studies, 6*(4), 402–433.

Goddard, R. D., Hoy, W. K., & Hoy, A. W. (2004). Collective efficacy beliefs: Theoretical developments, empirical evidence, and future directions. *Educational Researcher, 33*(3), 3–13.

Grant, L., & Langpap, C. (2019). Private provision of public goods by environmental groups. *Proceedings of the National Academy of Sciences, 116*(12), 5334–5340.

Gui, F., Tsai, C.-H., & Carroll, J. M. (2022). Community acknowledgment: Engaging community members in volunteer acknowledgment. *Proceedings of the ACM on Human-Computer Interaction, 6* (GROUP), 1–18.

Jo, J., Knearem, T., & Carroll, J. M. (2023). Coproducing support together: Sustain- able and reciprocal civic disaster relief during covid-19. *Proceedings of the ACM on Human-Computer Interaction, 7* (CSCW1), 1–25.

Jo, J., Knearem, T., Tsai, C.-H., & Carroll, J. M. (2021). Covid-19 kindness: Patterns of neighborly cooperation during a global pandemic. In *Proceedings of the 10th International Conference on Communities & Technologies-Wicked Problems in the Age of Tech*, (pp. 1–14).

Knearem, T., Jo, J., Alliyu, O., & Carroll, J. M. (2024). Solidarity not charity! Empowering local communities for disaster relief during covid-19 through grassroots support. *Computer Supported Cooperative Work (CSCW), 1*, 46.

Knearem, T., Jo, J., & Carroll, J. M. (2021). Local community support for tangible food aid during covid-19. In *Companion publication of the 2021 Conference on Computer Supported Cooperative Work and Social Computing*, (pp. 104–107).

Knearem, T., Jo, J., Tsai, C.-H., & Carroll, J. M. (2021). Making space for support: An exploratory analysis of pandemic-response mutual aid platforms. In *Proceedings of the 10th International Conference on Communities & Technologies-Wicked Problems in the Age of Tech* (pp. 38–43).

Knearem, T., Jo, J., Tsai, C.-H., & Carroll, J. M. (2022). Making community beliefs and capacities visible through care-mongering during covid-19. *Proceedings of the ACM on Human-Computer Interaction, 6* (GROUP), 1–19.

Knearem, T., Wang, X., Wan, J., & Carroll, J. M. (2019). Crafting in a community of practice: Resource sharing as key in supporting creativity. In *Proceedings of the 2019 Conference on Creativity and Cognition*, (pp. 83–94).

Lee, S., Reddie, M., Tsai, C.-H., Beck, J., Rosson, M. B., & Carroll, J. M. (2020). The emerging professional practice of remote sighted assistance for people with visual impairments. In *Proceedings of the 2020 CHI Conference on Human Factors in Computing Systems* (pp. 1–12).

Lin, Y.-F., Li, N., Huang, W.-H., Ecsedy, K., Feinberg, M. E., Teti, D., & Carroll, J. M. (2024). ultimately we re togetherâĹ⁻: Understanding new parents experiences of co-parenting. *Proceedings of the ACM on Human-Computer Interaction, 8* (CSCW2), 1–25.

Little, K. E., Hayashi, M., & Liang, S. (2016). Community-based groundwater monitoring network using a citizen-science approach. *Groundwater, 54*(3), 317–324.

Maslow, A. H. (1967). A theory of metamotivation: The biological rooting of the value-life. *Journal of Humanistic Psychology, 7*(2), 93–127.

References

McKellar, L. V., Pincombe, J. I., & Henderson, A. M. (2006). Insights from Australian parents into educational experiences in the early postnatal period. *Midwifery, 22*(4), 356–364.

McLeod, S. (2007). Maslow s hierarchy of needs. *Simply Psychology, 1* (1–18).

Ostrom, E. (1996). Crossing the great divide: Coproduction, synergy, and development. *World Development, 24*(6), 1073–1087.

Perren, S., Von Wyl, A., & B urgin, D., Simoni, H., & Von Klitzing, K. (2005). Depressive symptoms and psychosocial stress across the transition to parenthood: Associations with parental psychopathology and child difficulty. *Journal of Psychosomatic Obstetrics & Gynecology, 26*(3), 173–183.

Pew Research Center. (2015). Family support in graying societies. Retrieved March 17, 2024, from https://www.pewresearch.org/social-trends/2015/05/21/family-support-in-graying-societies/

Ramchandani, P. G., Domoney, J., Sethna, V., Psychogiou, L., Vlachos, H., & Murray, L. (2013). Do early father infant interactions predict the onset of exter-nalising behaviours in young children? findings from a longitudinal cohort study. *Journal of Child Psychology and Psychiatry, 54*(1), 56–64.

Sandbulte, J., Tsai, C.-H., & Carroll, J. M. (2021). Family s health: Opportunities for non-collocated intergenerational families collaboration on healthy living. *International Journal of Human-Computer Studies, 146*, 102559.

Silvertown, J. (2009). A new dawn for citizen science. *Trends in Ecology & Evolution, 24*(9), 467–471.

Stevens, M., Vitos, M., Altenbuchner, J., Conquest, G., Lewis, J., & Haklay, M. (2014). Taking participatory citizen science to extremes. *IEEE Pervasive Computing, 13*(2), 20–29.

Stuifbergen, M. C., Van Delden, J. J., & Dykstra, P. A. (2008). The implications of today s family structures for support giving to older parents. *Ageing & Society, 28*(3), 413–434.

Sun, R. (2016). Intergenerational age gaps and a family member s well-being: A family systems approach. *Journal of Intergenerational Relationships, 14*(4), 320–337.

Tan, J., Jin, F., & Dennis, A. (2020). Attention or appreciation? The impact of feedback on online volunteering.

Twenge, J. M., Campbell, W. K., & Foster, C. A. (2003). Parenthood and marital satisfaction: A meta-analytic review. *Journal of Marriage and Family, 65*(3), 574–583.

Wakschlag, L. S., & Hans, S. L. (1999). Relation of maternal responsiveness during infancy to the development of behavior problems in high-risk youths. *Developmental Psychology, 35*(2), 569.

Webber, T., Durbin, D.-A., & D Innocenzio, A. (2020). Volunteers sew masks for health workers facing shortages. https://abcnews.go.com/US/wireStory/volunteers-sew-masks-health-workers-facing-shortages-69764445

Wenger, E. (2011). Communities of practice: A brief introduction.

Winterich, K. P., Mittal, V., & Aquino, K. (2013). When does recognition increase charitable behavior? Toward a moral identity-based model. *Journal of Marketing, 77*(3), 121–134.

World Health Organization. (2020). Timeline of who s response to covid-19. Retrieved March 17, 2024, from https://www.who.int/news/item/29-06-2020-covidtimeline

Discussion

3.1 Coproducing Care is a Good Way to Work

Traditional measures of care reside in relatively static and top-down responsibility assignment, where the recipient passively receives care from the provider. Such assignment is understandable in systems of custodial care; the recipient may be unable to reciprocate or perhaps to take initiative at all. But in many cases, top-down administration of care is not forced, and there are downsides of placing care recipients in a passive position where the power differential between provider and recipient is sharp and pervades the interaction. A lessened sense of control and autonomy leads to decreased self-efficacy (Bandura et al., 1999) and self-determination (Spade, 2020), which may downgrade the overall quality of care.

For instance, physicians' objectification of patients and their sole focus on physical dysfunctions resulted in overlooking patients' distress and the habits that may perpetuate their disease (Haque & Waytz, 2012; Trifiletti et al., 2014; Vaes & Muratore, 2013). Similarly, many patients who are dependent on physicians or their family for care can feel helplessness and guilt due to their increased dependency, which over time was found to negatively affect self-esteem and physical functioning (Senescu, 1963). Custodial healthcare systems that focus merely on patients' physical functioning promote dependency on others for treatment, which can limit the overall quality of both mental health and physical care. In the case discussed in Sect. 2.6, prior to joining to coproduce disaster relief, citizens experienced feelings of guilt and helplessness confined to their homes, viewing themselves solely as aid recipients in contrast to healthcare workers on the frontlines to treat overwhelming numbers of COVID-19 infectants.

Our cases emphasize that the coproduction of care can intervene and restructure traditional custodial care to benefit both stakeholders in caring (care recipients and care providers) placing them in **a reciprocal and equitable relationship**. The boundary between care recipients and providers is blurred in coproduction, and all stakeholders are necessary for producing care. When engaging in care activities as equitable parties, stakeholders can **feel a sense of control** in producing care because they perceive that they can make an impact on decisions and contribute to their own care production.

In the shopping examples in Sect. 2.3, the sighted and non-sighted individuals who engaged in collaborative shopping played their respective roles, which contributed to shared care regardless of their physical abilities. They each had a sense of control over the shopping tasks and their strengths were leveraged. They were regarded as indispensable parties to make the task more efficient and complement the partner's roles, which they appreciated with respect. The examples contrast with conventional custodial care situations where families or friends complete the entire shopping task for people with visual impairments. Care is not mutual but unidirectional, depriving people with physical limitations of a sense of control in a routine task, which makes them heavily dependent on their family or friends.

In the family health care scenario, care between parents and children were not successfully delivered when perceived as intrusive, encroaching upon family members' independence. This resulted from one party assuming their role relegated to care recipient, while the other was considered a caregiver. To foster effective care provision, a fundamental shift in way of thinking one another's role was needed, where both parties redefine themselves and the other as reciprocal caregivers, care partners.

In the earlier NHS depression scenarios outlined by Cahn and Gray (2013), patients no longer passively received care and treatment from mental health professionals. Patients collaboratively self-managed their care with similar others which attenuated their depressive symptoms and increased confidence and self-esteem (Repper & Carter, 2011). Capabilities to improve mental health status were no longer the sole possessions of mental health professionals in the NHS scenarios.

In the example of community-based water monitoring introduced in Sect. 2.4, citizens collaborated with scientists and government authorities to monitor water quality in their region. Water quality monitoring plays a critical role in safeguarding the health of both communities and watersheds. However, the traditional approach taken by government agencies, though essential, exemplifies custodial care and comes with limitations. The restricted allocation of resources to these agencies often results in inadequate watershed monitoring, leading to temporal and spatial knowledge gaps regarding the health of our water resources (Kinchy et al., 2016). Citizen science helps address this gap and facilitates coproduction of community health through environmental monitoring. In our study, citizens had their own voice and autonomy in ensuring water quality through water monitoring activities. Participants of community-based water monitoring activities were on an equal plane, regardless of their status as local residents, scientists, or government officials, and collaboratively improved the local resources that they shared. In the design hackathon workshops, citizens' voices were equally respected as others' and regarded as one of the autonomous stakeholders regarding safe water.

In the example of community fridges discussed in Sect. 2.6, they effectively supplemented the limitations of formal food assistance by involving individuals who had firsthand experience with such aid. Rather than being seen as passive beneficiaries in need of food support, they were recognized as valuable contributors with insights into how grassroots initiatives could effectively complement formal aid programs. Through their involvement in producing food support, these individuals gained more autonomy within the food assistance system and developed a stronger sense of agency. Community fridges thus incorporated the perspectives and values of those directly using the commons.

The examples we discussed demonstrate how coproducing care can foster agency, responsibility taking and equality among engaged individuals, who are interdependent with one another without having one side dependent on the other and whose unique values are essential in building care. In this sense, we argue that participants in coproducing care can attain self-determination, which encompasses autonomy (a sense of control), competence (feeling effective in one's activity), and relatedness (a sense of connection to others) (Ryan & Deci, 2000). Achieving self-determination can enhance well-being and mental health, contributing to salutogenetic health. With the lens of Maslow's hierarchy of needs (Maslow, 1967), while custodial care can satisfy fundamental needs represented at the bottoms of the hierarchy (e.g., food, water, resources, health, and security), coproducing care goes beyond, addressing higher-level needs by fostering a sense of belonging with other stakeholders, esteem from heightened status and recognition, and self-actualization from effectively exerting one's potential through producing care.

Graeber (2012) suggests that true exchange or reciprocity requires that all parties involved hold similar status, engaging in ongoing interactions to achieve balance. If parties hold nonequivalent or hierarchical statuses, interactions are governed less by mutual exchange or reciprocity but rather by established traditions, habits, or societal norms. Graeber's emphasis on the need for equivalent status among parties for true reciprocity can be applied to the concept of coproduced care by advocating for a shift from hierarchical, custodial care models practiced by habits to more equitable, participatory ones.

3.2 The Spectrum of Coproduction

The impact and importance of coproduction in various disciplines has introduced various definitions and variations of coproduction. For instance, the prominent visionaries of coproduction, Ostrom and Cahn, primarily focused on two somewhat different arenas. Ostrom focused on the importance of reciprocal services in public administration, and Cahn's view of coproduction resides predominantly in empowering marginalized communities.

Glynos and Speed (2012) also add to this array of defining and distinguishing coproduction services and outcomes. They view coproduction to be either additive or transformative based on the outcome of the activity. Although they don't explicitly mention whether additive and transformative coproduction are dichotomous or not, their focus on incorporating timebanks in healthcare transformatively appears to be categorical. In contrast, just like soft and hard services, used by Brudney and England (1983), tend to have a fuzzy boundary, we see the additive and transformative classification of coproduction as more of a spectrum than a binary classification.

In our analysis, we used the additive and transformative models to analyze various coproduction activities in the case studies and noticed that coproduction is usually a mixture of both additive and transformative. We found that the roles of initiators and joiners in the coproduction activities were variable and often changed in different situations. This variability in role changes makes additive and transformative two tendencies in a spectrum of coproduction. Hence, to the extent that it is a spectrum, it isn't categorical but a matter of more or less. For instance, in Cahn's example of a person suffering from depression, the person becomes an instrument of their own treatment by helping and socializing with other people. Similarly, in Ostrom's policing example, role change in the community transformed the safety of the community. Coproduction and role changes between police and citizens can both add to the community safety and harmony, and also transform the community relationships and functions.

We created a conceptual model to better exhibit our analysis of the spectrum of coproduction for care, with respect to the traditional custodial form of care (see Fig. 3.1). In the traditional custodial form of care, the provider holds the capacity and skills to deliver care to the receiver, who in turn recognizes the care being provided. Hence, in a custodial care model, flow of care from provider to receiver is unidirectional. Custodial care is to directly provide professional effective instrumental support that the one-directional management by the caregivers, such as institutional physical and mental healthcare. On the other hand, coproducing care is a bidirectional model where the roles of provider and receiver are transformed to that of an initiator and joiner. Both of these new roles hold capacity, skills and recognition, since care is coproduced through mutual and reciprocal activities. Both initia-

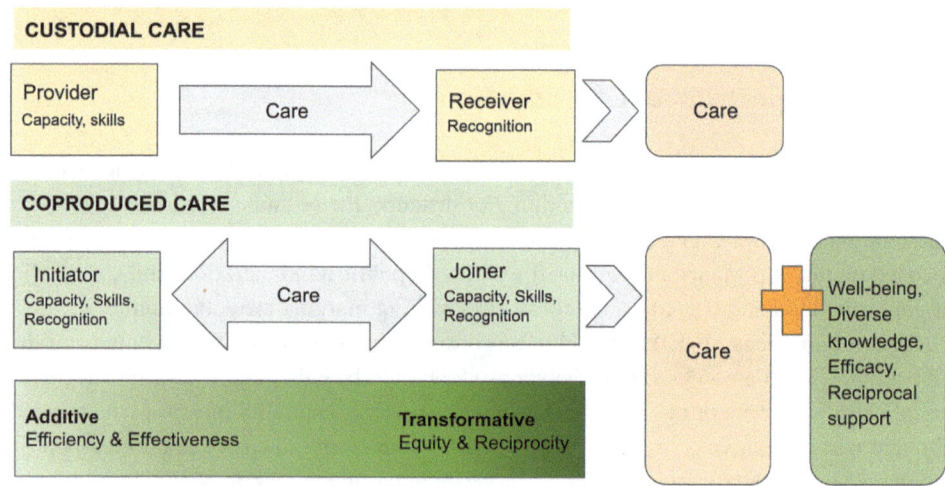

Fig. 3.1 Contrasting custodial and coproduced care

3.2 The Spectrum of Coproduction

tors and joiners are active participants in coproduction activities, hence the outcome of this care model includes both provision of care and mutual dependence. In our coproducing care model, both the initiator and joiner are equal contributors in the reciprocal care activities, and everyone involved is equally empowered by the outcome. Whereas, in unidirectional custodial care, only the provider feels efficacious.

Our case study analysis also bolsters the above argument for a spectrum of coproduction. For instance, in the case of water quality monitoring, citizen science initiatives were both additive and transformative. They were additive because they added to civic and institutional water monitoring efforts, and they were transformative because citizen participation created synergy in the community by coproducing scientific knowledge, environmental health, and enhanced social capital.

In a family unit, care provided by adult children to elderly parents is additive when accepted by the parents, yet it also changes family roles and thus transforms towards care reciprocity between family members as they become active partners. In the scenario of co-parenting, the behavior that one parent makes extra efforts to support another parent both physically and mentally not only creates additive coproduction of having their baby grow in a more supportive and resourceful environment but also subsequently transforms their family bonds to be closer as they become more experienced regarding communicating with their partners and understanding what their partners need.

Similarly, in the case of community acknowledgment, the act of thanking local community groups was additive as it helped increase the morale of community volunteers, in-turn increasing their productivity; and it was transformative because thank you card writing was beneficial to the volunteers as they felt that their hard work was acknowledged, their services' quality was assured, and the meaning of their work was enhanced. Moreover, from the thank-you note station activity, community members learned about local non-profit groups that they were previously unaware of.

In the case of citizen-based disaster relief efforts, they were additive in that they operated at double capacity in conjunction with existing formal relief groups (e.g., nonprofit organizations) to better combat long-lasting crises of the pandemic and food insecurity. It was transformative because they provided care to those who are often in role of providing support (e.g., frontline workers), marginalized populations also joined to coproduce relief efforts, and reshaped how individuals think about their responsibilities towards others in their community.

The spectrum of coproduction was also reflected in the beer brewing community. The role of initiators and joiners changed during knowledge exchange process, engendering new or unanticipated information that helped produce new knowledge and educate the participants, thereby transforming the beer brewing activity.

3.3 Synergy as a Defining Characteristic of Coproduction

Coproduction generates synergies between the parties involved (Ostrom, 1996) that strengthen social ties between participants (Chen et al., 2019). Previously, we have discussed how and why coproduction is more than just collaboration. However, the word coproduction has sometimes been used as a positive synonym for what is actually a *collaboration*. The primary difference between the two concepts is that collaboration can be synergistic, but it doesn't need to be, while synergy is a natural outcome of coproduction. Collaboration often takes the form of division of labor, with motivation being to reduce the workload on any one person and/or complete tasks efficiently. In contrast, coproduction goes beyond collaboration in that the parties complete their tasks collaboratively yet also achieve additional outcomes unrelated to the core tasks, such as positive effects on personal well-being. One way to look at this is that the combined effect of the parties coming together is greater than merely completing the task or reaching a mutually stated goal. In this way, synergy differentiates coproduction from collaboration.

The cases we elaborated on in Sect. 2.1 provide evidence for the synergetic outcomes of care coproduction. When adult children cooked a meal with their elderly parents, their endeavor not only resulted in a healthy meal, but also an opportunity to care for each other. When parents supported their partners in childrearing tasks, they not only took care of their child's well-being but also their relationships. Also, the closer relationship, in turn, fosters further mutual support and communication between the couple. People with visual impairments both initiated and joined in shopping experiences. They were able to complete their shopping lists, but had the added benefits of feeling valued and respected by their sighted companions. The older adults who engaged in water monitoring accomplished the task of collecting baseline data, while also enjoying each other's company and getting physical exercise. Acknowledging the good works of others in the local community resulted in volunteers' feeling gratitude. Community members also learned something about their community when writing cards to thank local organizations for their work. Finally, when hobbyist home brewers shared their brewing knowledge with other brewers, they helped solve problems while at the same time gained unexpected knowledge from other members' experiences. The synergy between these participants, not the task or stated goal, is what led to the variety of care outcomes illustrated in the case studies.

Engagements across the spectrum of coproduction may be influenced by the relationships between parties. Some of the relationships in our cases were institutionalized (e.g., marriage, family structure), while others were not (e.g., hobbyists, volunteers, citizens). Familial relationships may provide the circumstances and structure for frequent coproduction opportunities to occur. In addition, the roles in family relationships (e.g., parent/child, husband/wife) may lend themselves as trustworthy, thereby increasing the chances for care coproduction. This is transformative in that it leverages and strengthens existing familial bonds and relationships in a new way. However, institutionalized relationships are not a requirement for coproducing care, as was illustrated by the cases of the water monitoring volunteers and home brewers who engaged in coproduction across the spectrum in non-institutionalized relationships.

Our cases suggest that engagement in an initial care coproduction is oftentimes enough to encourage future participation in additional coproduction. Over time, repeated coproduction activities build a cycle of coproducing care, in which the well-being outcomes that both the initiators and joiners experience are personally satisfying enough to create mutual care for each other which precedes additional coproduction. In line with Klinenberg (2018)'s assertion that social cohesion is cultivated through continuous and repeated interactions, along with collective engagement in achieving common goals, regular engagement in coproducing care enables parties to maintain the care relationship. This, in turn, strengthens their mutual commitment to one another's well-being.

For instance, those who participated in COVID-19 disaster relief activities redefined their capabilities and responsibilities towards neighbors, added relief efforts to care for a broader range of populations in their local communities, and were committed to persisting in their caring activities beyond the pandemic era. Community fridges facilitated regular interactions among local members, some of whom were previously strangers, engaging in casual conversations, joining in community events, and initiating further support activities. These interactions and common goals towards alleviating food insecurity and waste issues strengthened social ties, fostering mutual trust. Local members grew to believe that their neighbors were there for everyday support and that they could overcome community challenges via a tightly-knit neighborhood network. Our cases suggest that moving from the less-committal additive side of the spectrum towards transformative coproduction is built on a foundation of commitment to regular interaction, in which the outcomes of the coproduction produce fulfilling well-being outcomes.

Researchers in our own interdisciplinary community of HCI (Human Computer Interaction), and specifically CSCW (Computer-Supported Cooperative Work), have investigated the key concepts of cooperation and collaboration since the 1980s (Ciolfi et al., 2023; Olsson et al., 2020). Yet the concept of coproduction, well recognized in many social science contexts, is almost never mentioned, nor is the specific importance of enabling and recognizing contributions of all participants in order to coproduce effective and equitable social outcomes. We reported in Chapter 1 a survey of recent studies of care from the HCI/CSCW community, and the very limited extent to which non-custodial care was represented. We suggest that coproduction should be added to the pantheon of cooperation and collaboration.

3.4 Future Implications

How can we better incorporate the principle of coproduction in our approach to designing care systems as researchers? This section delves into the implications for research practices and practical design strategies that encourage the coproduction of care, insights drawn from our case studies. We discovered that coproduction of care can be realized through:

(1) recognition of stakes; (2) recognition of individual contributions; (3) recognition of resources. We will discuss how these aspects of recognition manifest in our case studies.

3.4.1 Making Different Stakes Salient

Receiving care is bidirectional in the coproduction of care, to *initiators* and to *joiners*, where their requirements are more variable than in custodial care. These combined and complex requirements make it essential to identify the perspectives and roles of *initiators* and *joiners* in advance and constantly throughout the care system. It should be noted that within traditional care systems, the voice of care recipients is often not heard but rather assumed by care providers. Therefore, initial and ongoing communications among all parties are necessary to have their voice heard and to have complex requirements met.

For instance, we presented an example of a family situation where the young adult child wanted to help the elderly parent by writing a diet plan without taking into consideration the parent's beliefs and thoughts about healthy living. Although the adult child's intention was positive since it sought to support the parent's healthy eating habit, still the parent dismissed the child's attempt to show care. In contrast, elderly parents wanted to care for their children although adult children felt that they were hovering over them. In these situations, we argue that acknowledging individual differences and leveraging diverse insights on health may contribute to a more effective strategy to promote cooperation on health within families. One practical example is our prior study in Sandbulte et al. (2021) where we examined family members' and friends' engagement and awareness on healthy behaviors while living apart through a technological intervention. We learned that bringing family members together to cooperate equally as active partners would enable the synergistic effect of coproduction.

In the case of co-parenting, one parent may not feel satisfied with the childcare distribution, yet is hesitant to discuss with their partner due to the fear of tension or hurting the partner's feelings. In scenarios where one party feels hesitant to state their needs, designers could support respectful communication between partners by offering structured conversation prompts and scaffolding that reduce the fear of emotional harm. Prior work in computer-mediated communication has shown that AI-mediated structured dialogues can foster constructive (**exchangeschan2017wakey**). Building on this, designers might leverage large language models (LLMs) to help suggest the refinement of potentially sensitive messages into more considerate language. For instance, AI could suggest alternative phrasings based on established communication frameworks like John Gottman's "Four Horsemen" approach, which guides couples toward healthier interaction patterns by encouraging the use of soft starts, appreciation, and personal responsibility (Gottman et al., 2008).

Systems for care coproduction should embrace adaptability, evolving based on collaborative inputs. From our community-based water monitoring initiative, we learned that participatory approaches, such as hackathons, can serve as forums to incorporate diverse perspectives of stakeholders. The hackathon facilitated knowledge exchange but also transformed residents from passive beneficiaries of water monitoring groups to active contributors, sharing their opinions on various problems and presenting design scenarios that reflect problems and solutions at a micro level, say, a resident home or neighborhood. The hackathon fostered their deeper communal engagement and collective sense of responsibility around their watershed. Our case study reflects that hackathons can facilitate coproduction through collective ideation and co-creation of solutions, also allowing researchers to embrace the stakes of involved parties to better design systems for coproducing care.

Engaging all relevant stakeholders is crucial for effective coproduction, yet people are prone to interact with individuals with more similar backgrounds to themselves. As HCI researchers, we must always be mindful that technology-mediated interventions, such as care coproduction, can inadvertently exclude individuals with limited access to information technology. In fact, broad access for most people to digital devices, including internet connectivity, and high digital literacy has the effect of penalizing people with limited digital opportunities even further.

To foster more transformative care, it is essential to proactively include those typically seen as care recipients. Section 2.6 presented a scenario where digitally disadvantaged individuals declined donated laptops. This example illustrates that integrating them into care coproduction requires more than just providing technological access. We argue that designing for transformative care coproduction require careful considerations of who we design for, who could be excluded from the designs, and how they could be engaged via a deep understanding of their stakes and viewpoints.

3.4.2 Making Contributions Visible

Coproduction of care may not always involve all relevant people jointly performing a given task simultaneously. Care recipient in a custodial care system can conversely give care to usual care providers simply through recognizing their work. Some care givers in our society are invisible and undervalued as their work is not so powerful or taken for granted (Star & Strauss, 1999). We can provide care for those workers by increasing their awareness and showing gratitude for their work.

In the co-parenting example discussed in Sect. 2.2, parents bolstered their partners' self-esteem by valuing the recognition of effort and competence, seeing trust from their partners as vital in parenting. This recognition of their efforts by their partners played a significant role in enhancing their confidence. However, it is sometimes difficult for parents to show appreciation explicitly. Making parents aware of the appreciation from their partners in a way that is comfortable for both parties would be a good way to maintain coproduction. While words of affirmation are direct and easily understood, parents may prefer to express appreciation and love through alternative, less verbal forms (Chapman, 2010). Designers could explore ways to support these diverse expressions, such as acts of service or shared activities, by making them more visible and meaningful without being overly explicit. Subtle design cues or ambient feedback mechanisms could help ensure these gestures are recognized and appreciated, while still respecting the parents' communication style and comfort levels. For example, leveraging a done list of the childcare tracking apps to track a partner's contributions to childcare, such as through visual logs or gentle summaries, can help increase mutual awareness and foster appreciation (Lin et al., 2025). Prior work has found that highlighting a husband's caregiving efforts might help the wife recognize and value his involvement more consciously, potentially strengthening their emotional connection (Jo et al., 2020). Designers could explore subtle, non-competitive ways to surface these contributions to encourage gratitude and shared understanding.

In the community appreciation example, local community members, who indirectly benefited from non-profit groups, were not so aware of their efforts. In our previous study (Gui et al., 2022), we designed and distributed the thank you note stations to first raise awareness of those non-profit groups and second to provide activities for community members to appreciate them and take part in the caregiving process. We achieved the first goal by presenting non-profit groups' activities in a slideshow that allowed community members to recognize these community efforts. To achieve the second goal, we invited community members to take action at the thank you stations by writing thank you cards. Through writing thank you cards, community members, who usually are care receivers became caregivers showing appreciations towards non-profit volunteers. As the non-profits receive care through these appreciations, they are more likely to sustain their volunteer work which benefits more community members. In our example, the thank-you note station worked as a tool to make contributions of invisible caregivers visible and to let community members generate care by expressing their gratitude.

In the disaster relief example described in Sect. 2.6, individuals who received gratitude expressed their thanks to those who had shown appreciation, creating a reciprocal cycle of care coproduction within the community. Our participant running a local restaurant prepared meals for frontline workers as a gesture of appreciation for their high-risk efforts. In turn, frontline workers visited her restaurant to express their gratitude for her recognition of their hard work, supporting her business by purchasing meals.

Our case studies reveal that expressing gratitude serves as a moral incentive, fostering a cycle of prosocial behavior (McCullough et al., 2002). Similar initiatives can be implemented in various contexts to raise awareness and reciprocate care to care initiators, benefiting everyone involved in the care ecosystem. For instance, integrating a virtual space for acknowledging care initiators into online platforms for coproducing care could enhance such appreciation. In personal settings, e.g., co-parenting, a dedicated space for expressing gratitude could lead to more frequent exchanges of acknowledgement and increase perceived genuineness. In collective settings, public acknowledgment of care initiators can motivate them to persist in producing care, recognizing that their endeavors matter and is impactful, and enable care recipients to join caring work by reciprocating care for initiators. Public acknowledgment can also elevate the visibility of care work to third parties, potentially

3.4.3 Making Better Use of Resources

In a custodial care system, care is unidirectional, and resources of those who receive care are under-leveraged. Within coproduction of care, where none of the parties merely receive care, it is integral to identify those resources under-leveraged in a custodial care system. Designs should not be rigid but instead be open to encompass all capabilities. When potentials of all parties are realized, the outcome and quality of care can be maximized. Abilities of these under-leveraged and marginalized people can be recognized once their roles are not predefined (Glynos & Speed, 2012), but are determined in accordance with their abilities.

Previous work suggests similar ideas, calling for emphasis on ability rather than disabilities (Liu et al., 2016) and deficits, such as ability-based design (Wobbrock et al., 2011) in accessible computing literature, the strength-based approach in social work studies (Saleebey, 1996), and the asset-based approach in community development literature (Kretzmann & McKnight, 1993). Within the asset-based approach, assets are defined as "strengths, attributes, and resources that can be brought into relevance to satisfy the inherent tensions between a member of a population's needs, their understood or experienced aspirations, and the structural limitations of the system" (Gautam & Tatar, 2022). In a parallel vein, in the community fridge example, individuals benefiting from government food assistance programs actively participated in managing community fridges, guiding the fridges to complement the limitations of government programs (e.g., limited operation time, limited access to fresh food). Without their participation in coproducing food support, the limitations of government programs in fulfilling needs of individuals experiencing food insecurity might have remained unrecognized and unmet by community fridge groups.

Section 2.3 discusses examples where people with visual impairment (PVI) collaborate with their family members during grocery shopping. In custodial care settings, PVI are predefined in a passive role, and are taken care of when their family members go shopping on their behalf. They can be marginalized and excluded from everyday activities, such as shopping trips. However, in our examples, their abilities to determine which products to purchase, provide a sense of direction, and interpersonal communication skills contribute to more efficient shopping were identified and fully utilized.

In our example of collaborative beer brewing (Knearem et al., 2018), professional brewers and home brewers were placed in equal positions to contribute their knowledge during the collaborative brewing activity. The role of sharing knowledge on beer brewing was not confined only to professional brewers. Home brewers were welcomed to share their knowledge and to participate in creating richer learning experiences, sometimes even leading the discussion in place of professional brewers. These enhanced learning opportunities would not have been possible if the environment was rigid and they were not allowed to intervene. In the collaborative beer brewing example, all involved parties were given a chance to produce care in an atmosphere where anyone could spontaneously join and lead the group.

As we are likely to be entrenched in prevalent custodial care, recognizing and utilizing under-leveraged capacities necessitates thinking out of the box. Here, we suggest that identifying and documenting skills and resources through asset mapping, inspired from the asset-based community development approach, offer a practical framework for capacity building and action. Asset mapping is used to uncover tangible and intangible assets (e.g., personal skills) within a community (Kretzmann & McKnight, 1996). Beyond merely documenting an asset inventory, the mapping process involves interpreting these assets to consider how they can meet collective goals, identify collaboration opportunities, and determine ways to strengthen these assets for community empowerment. For researchers designing to coproduce care, this approach can be applied at either collective or individual levels, depending on stakeholder relationships, to discover under-leveraged capacities. Furthermore, integrating asset mapping tools into systems for coproducing care can make visible under-leveraged capacities of involved parties, thereby empowering marginalized individuals who are often regarded as care receivers in the custodial care model to participate actively in coproduction. Recognition of their capabilities not only increases their voice, but it also augments the quality of produced care.

3.5 Limitations and Future Work

Our cases suggest that coproduction of care can take place in everyday interactions, and can be beneficial for well being. However, several limitations should be noted. First, our cases centered on relatively informal family and community-based care interactions. However, care can occur in many social contexts. Ostrom's coproduction research investigated public administration contexts. Her work showed how the citizen relationship with government could be improved by adapting coproduction of care to social services. Ostrom's example of the synergy of solidarity generated from police and citizens encountering one another in the street and recognizing their shared commitment to improving community safety. This example is inspiring but it raises further questions: Where is the line, and how can we draw the line, between responsible citizen engagement and misguided vigilantism or interference with official police activity?

Other examples can be drawn from custodial care in institutional contexts, such as healthcare and education. We think that patient and student agency should be more typical in such contexts. But we also see that these contexts are much more complex than informal family and community contexts, and often cannot rely on a pre-existing stock of trust and commitment. For example, patients and students can vary significantly in their willingness and even in their capabilities to be responsible agents in their own care. Indeed, such variation can itself lead institutions to favor custodial approaches. But a more salutogenic way of framing the challenge is to ask how much self-agency and responsibility is effective for each person.

3.5 Limitations and Future Work

For example, we know that some people in hospitals will not recover, but this should not preclude their opportunity to contribute to their own care. Rather, they should participate in ways and to the extent that doing so coproduces better care and a better care experience for them. We do not know how to do this.

Second, our cases are taken from a Western context; we investigated the coproduction of care in families and communities primarily from the United States. This provides a starting point for future work to broaden the scope of care coproduction to include examples from other cultures, other countries and other regions. Indeed, the prior we built upon, by Edgar Cahn and Elinor Ostrom, was also carried out primarily in the United States. Our cases also were biased in that our participants wanted to take responsibility, to share control, and to participate reliably in their various activities. In presenting our work at various research events, we have several times encountered shock and disapproval at the proposition that care could or should be coproduced. One attitude we have encountered is that coproducing care implicitly devalues caregiving, though it is more accurate to say that it reduces the singular authority and responsibility of the caregiver.

The assumption that a caregiver is in charge of care is one of several cultural views that might be problematic for people interested in adopting coproduction of care. Thus, people can understand care as requiring and depending upon a caregiver. They may regard being asked or expected to be involved at all in the details of their care as an indicator of a failure of that care. People might see care as a category of interaction that is always paid for, or more generally, provided as a professional service. They might feel disrespected if it is suggested that they can play a role in care interactions. Future research could explore coproduction adoption and practice on the basis of individual or culture differences.

Third, although we use transformative and additive coproduction classification to analyze our case studies, there are other taxonomies of coproduction such as "hard services" and "soft services" (Brudney & England, 1983) that include all kinds of service coproductions. Soft services include areas that require direct participation such as education and healthcare. On the other hand, hard services such as police work and emergency response do not require direct citizen participation, but such participation can facilitate more successful and transformative services, as described by Ostrom. Our investigation did not include instances of hard services in Brudney's classification, but future work should do that.

Our study showed that coproducing care is a good way to work, but in order to clearly explain how it works in different situations, a more comprehensive model is needed. We view coproduction across an additive/transformative spectrum, and describe how a system of coproducing care system could apply dynamically. We compare our way of looking at care with custodial care to show its strengths, and identify the essential elements in this framework such as reciprocity and individual capability. However, in order to better understand the coproduction in care practice and be able to have it tailored for various scenarios, future studies could further address its fundamental principles, boundaries, and working mechanisms with advanced theoretical models.

3.6 Conclusion

We noticed patterns of reciprocal caring across a set of our investigations into relatively intimate and small scale social systems. It was striking to us that coproduced care can be better for all participants in care relationships - caring is amplified through reciprocity and recognition when participants are both care givers and cared for, and social roles and relationships among participants expand and develop in nuanced ways that facilitate providing and accepting care.

We are mindful that our analysis requires further confirmation and development, and that traditional conceptions of custodial care are still relevant and important. On the other hand, active and reciprocal care arrangements may be a path toward more and better care for everyone, and for care that emphasizes participation that enriches and expands human growth, instead of merely mitigating deficits.

References

Bandura, A., Freeman, W. H., & Lightsey, R. (1999). Self-efficacy: The exercise of control.

Brudney, J. L., & England, R. E. (1983). Toward a definition of the coproduction concept. *Public Administration Review*, 59–65.

Cahn, E. S., & Gray, C. (2013). Co-production from a normative perspective. In *New public governance, the third sector, and co-production* (pp. 129–144). Routledge.

Chapman, G. (2010). *The five love languages: The secret to love that lasts*. Chicago, IL.

Chen, J., Hanrahan, B. V., & Carroll, J. M. (2019). Withshare: A mobile application to support community coproduction activities. *International Journal of Mobile Human Computer Interaction (IJMHCI)*, *11*(1), 40–61.

Ciolfi, L., Lewkowicz, M., & Schmidt, K. (2023). Computer-supported cooperative work. In *Handbook of human computer interaction* (pp. 1–26). Springer.

Gautam, A., & Tatar, D. (2022). Empowering participation within structures of dependency. In *Proceedings of the Participatory Design Conference 2022* (Vol. 1, pp. 75–86).

Glynos, J., & Speed, E. (2012). Varieties of co-production in public services: Time banks in a UK health policy context. *Critical Policy Studies*, *6*(4), 402–433.

Gottman, J. M., et al. (2008). Gottman method couple therapy. *Clinical Handbook of Couple Therapy*, *4*(8), 138–164.

Graeber, D. (2012). Debt: The first 5000 years. Penguin UK.

Gui, F., Tsai, C.-H., & Carroll, J. M. (2022). Community acknowledgment: Engaging community members in volunteer acknowledgment. *Proceedings of the ACM on Human-Computer Interaction*, *6*(GROUP), 1–18.

Haque, O. S., & Waytz, A. (2012). Dehumanization in medicine: Causes, solutions, and functions. *Perspectives on Psychological Science*, *7*(2), 176–186.

Jo, E., Toombs, A. L., Gray, C. M., & Hong, H. (2020). Understanding parent- ing stress through co-designed self-trackers. In: Proceedings of the 2020 CHI Conference on Human Factors in Computing Systems (pp. 1–13).

Karau, S. J., & Williams, K. D. (1993). Social loafing: A meta-analytic review and theoretical integration. *Journal of Personality and Social Psychology*, *65*(4), 681.

References

Kinchy, A., Parks, S., & Jalbert, K. (2016). Fractured knowledge: Mapping the gaps in public and private water monitoring efforts in areas affected by shale gas development. *Environment and Planning C: Government and Policy, 34*(5), 879–899.

Klinenberg, E. (2018). Palaces for the people: How social infrastructure can help fight inequality, polarization, and the decline of civic life. Crown.

Knearem, T., Wang, X., Wan, J., & Carroll, J. M. (2019). Crafting in a community of practice: Resource sharing as key in supporting creativity. Proceedings of the 2019 Conference on Creativity and Cognition (pp. 83–94).

Kretzmann, J., & McKnight, J. P. (1996). Assets-based community development. *Nat l Civic Rev, 85*, 23.

Kretzmann, J. P., & McKnight, J. (1993). Building communities from the inside out.

Lin, Y.-F., Li, X., Huang, W.-H., Prabavathi, C. P., Cai, J., & Carroll, J. M. (2025). Parental collaboration and closeness: Envisioning with new couple parents. arXiv:2505.22428.

Liu, P., Ding, X., & Gu, N. (2016). helping others makes me happy social in- teraction and integration of people with disabilities. In *Proceedings of the 19th ACM Conference on Computer-Supported Cooperative Work & Social Computing* (pp. 1596–1608).

Maslow, A. H. (1967). A theory of metamotivation: The biological rooting of the value-life. *Journal of Humanistic Psychology, 7*(2), 93–127.

McCullough, M. E., Emmons, R. A., & Tsang, J.-A. (2002). The grateful disposition: A conceptual and empirical topography. *Journal of Personality and Social Psychology, 82*(1), 112.

Olsson, T., Jarusriboonchai, P., & Wo zniak, P., Paasovaara, S., Väänänen, K., & Lucero, A. (2020). Technologies for enhancing collocated social interaction: Review of design solutions and approaches. *Computer Supported Cooperative Work (CSCW), 29*, 29–83.

Ostrom, E. (1996). Crossing the great divide: Coproduction, synergy, and development. *World Development, 24*(6), 1073–1087.

Repper, J., & Carter, T. (2011). A review of the literature on peer support in mental health services. *Journal of Mental Health, 20*(4), 392–411.

Ryan, R. M., & Deci, E. L. (2000). Self-determination theory and the facilitation of intrinsic motivation, social development, and well-being. *American Psychologist, 55*(1), 68.

Saleebey, D. (1996). The strengths perspective in social work practice: Extensions and cautions. *Social Work, 41*(3), 296–305.

Sandbulte, J., Tsai, C.-H., & Carroll, J. M. (2021). Working together in a phamily-space: Facilitating collaboration on healthy behaviors over distance. *Proceedings of the ACM on Human-Computer Interaction, 5*(CSCW1), 1–32.

Senescu, R. A. (1963). The development of emotional complications in the patient with cancer. *Journal of Chronic Diseases, 16*(7), 813–832.

Spade, D. (2020). Mutual aid: Building solidarity during this crisis (and the next). Verso Books.

Star, S. L., & Strauss, A. (1999). Layers of silence, arenas of voice: The ecology of visible and invisible work. *Computer Supported Cooperative Work (CSCW), 8*, 9–30.

Trifiletti, E., Di Bernardo, G. A., Falvo, R., & Capozza, D. (2014). Patients are not fully human: A nurse s coping response to stress. *Journal of Applied Social Psychology, 44*(12), 768–777.

Vaes, J., & Muratore, M. (2013). Defensive dehumanization in the medical practice: A cross-sectional study from a health care worker s perspective. *British Journal of Social Psychology, 52*(1), 180–190.

Wobbrock, J. O., Kane, S. K., Gajos, K. Z., Harada, S., & Froehlich, J. (2011). Ability-based design: Concept, principles and examples. *ACM Transactions on Accessible Computing (TACCESS), 3*(3), 1–27.